The Mindful Guide to Managing DIABETES

YOUR PATH TO REDUCING STRESS AND LIVING WELL

Joseph P. Napora, Ph.D.

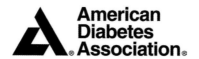

American Diabetes Association

Associate Publisher, Books, Abe Ogden; *Director, Book Operations,* Victor Van Beuren; *Managing Editor, Books,* John Clark; *Associate Director, Book Marketing,* Annette Reape; *Acquisitions Editor,* Jaclyn Konich; *Senior Manager, Book Editing,* Lauren Wilson; *Project Manager,* Wendy Martin-Shuma; *Composition,* Circle Graphics; *Cover Design,* Jenn French; *Printer,* Versa Press.

Printed in the United States of America

1 3 5 7 9 10 8 6 4 2

The suggestions and information contained in this publication are generally consistent with the *Standards of Medical Care in Diabetes* and other policies of the American Diabetes Association, but they do not represent the policy or position of the Association or any of its boards or committees. Reasonable steps have been taken to ensure the accuracy of the information presented. However, the American Diabetes Association cannot ensure the safety or efficacy of any product or service described in this publication. Individuals are advised to consult a physician or other appropriate health care professional before undertaking any diet or exercise program or taking any medication referred to in this publication. Professionals must use and apply their own professional judgment, experience, and training and should not rely solely on the information contained in this publication before prescribing any diet, exercise, or medication. The American Diabetes Association—its officers, directors, employees, volunteers, and members—assumes no responsibility or liability for personal or other injury, loss, or damage that may result from the suggestions or information in this publication.

Sean Petrie conducted the internal review of this book to ensure that it meets American Diabetes Association guidelines.

♾ The paper in this publication meets the requirements of the ANSI Standard Z39.48-1992 (permanence of paper).

ADA titles may be purchased for business or promotional use or for special sales. To purchase more than 50 copies of this book at a discount, or for custom editions of this book with your logo, contact the American Diabetes Association at the address below or at booksales@diabetes.org.

American Diabetes Association
2451 Crystal Drive, Suite 900
Arlington, VA 22202

DOI: 10.2337/9781580407106

Names: Napora, Joseph, author.
Title: The mindful guide to managing diabetes : your path to reducing stress and living well / Joseph P. Napora, PhD.
Description: Arlington : American Diabetes Association, [2019] | Includes bibliographical references and index.
Identifiers: LCCN 2019002778 | ISBN 9781580407106 (soft cover : alk. paper)
Subjects: LCSH: Diabetes--Popular works. | Diabetes--Treatment--Popular works. | Self-care, Health--Popular works.
Classification: LCC RC660.4 .N37 2019 | DDC 616.4/62--dc23
LC record available at https://lccn.loc.gov/2019002778

To Granny, my wife and very best friend.

And in memory of Martin, a dear friend
and a model of excellence.

Contents

ACKNOWLEDGMENTS

First, I want to express my gratitude to all of the individuals with diabetes who gave me inspiration and support over the years that I have worked in this field.

In addition, I am very grateful to Richard R. Rubin, to Chris Saudek of the Johns Hopkins Comprehensive Diabetes Center, to Bev Amsterdam Press of the Suburban Hospital Diabetes Center, Bethesda, MD, and to the many faculty and staff who gave me the opportunity and support in developing my work. Thanks, too, go to Marlys Rixey, Carrie Grady, Rachael L. Balter, and Nancy Glaser for their contributions to this endeavor.

Thanks also go to Victor Van Beuren of the American Diabetes Association. Victor has been an advocate of my work from the initial conversation we had about publishing the first edition, *Stress-Free Diabetes: Your Guide to Health and Happiness* (1). My appreciation goes to everyone who has played a role in the development, production, and promotion of the book, including Jaclyn Konich, Lauren Wilson, Wendy Martin-Shuma, and Annette Reape. Your commitment to making *The Mindful Guide to Managing Diabetes* the best it could be has been invaluable.

Once again, I am fortunate to have a loving family cheering me on during the process of writing this book. Their enthusiasm helped a lot. I have been blessed, too, by the spiritual guidance of Rabbis Steven Schwartz and Dana Saroken.

Last but not least, I am deeply appreciative of Linda, my wife and best friend, for her support, her patience, and her wise and tireless reaction to every written word.

FOREWORD

O dds are good that you've picked up this book because your personal experience has taught you that living well with diabetes is a lot more difficult when the everyday demands of life are driving you crazy. Not a big surprise, huh? Yes, stress and diabetes can be a toxic combination. And you no doubt know that the sources of stress are endless—your job, your family, your worries about money, your worries about your health, your lack of free time, and, of course, the demands and frustrations of living with diabetes. As denizens of the U.S. in the 21st century, we are all aswirl in a sea of stressful experiences, and it is too easy for our lives to grow more and more burdensome and out of control. Unrelenting stress can make it so much harder to give your diabetes the attention and care that it needs. My colleagues and I here at the Behavioral Diabetes Institute have been researching this problem for decades, and we now understand how chronic stress can lead to dangerously high blood glucose levels, both directly (due to stress-induced hormonal changes) and indirectly (due to stress-induced changes in behavior, such as overeating). But what on earth can you do about all this? You probably can't just up and move to some idyllic South Pacific island; even if you did, you'd probably just take many of your worries and concerns with you.

While you can't make all of the stresses in your life magically disappear, there are methods for directly addressing life stress and for alleviating the many stresses and aggravations of living with diabetes. So have hope; you can feel better and do better! One key solution is the application of mindfulness, and Dr. Joseph Napora does a terrific job of explaining the concept and showing you how a mindful approach can make a real difference in your life. In this book, he uses many real-life stories and examples to cut through the professional gobble-dygook (the unnecessary jargon that we psychologists are too prone to use) and gets to the heart of the issue. Also, being the kind and compassionate psychotherapist that he is, he does it all with real heart. Ready to start feeling better? Get ready for your adventure with Dr. Joe!

William H. Polonsky, PhD, CDE
President, Behavioral Diabetes Institute
Associate Clinical Professor,
University of California, San Diego

INTRODUCTION

C hances are that what you have learned about diabetes management has focused on diet, exercise, medication, and checking your blood glucose levels—certainly four essential aspects of effective glucose management. However, you may not know that controlling stress is a significant factor in managing diabetes.

Keeping the stress of diabetes and of life in general at a minimum, an essential for managing diabetes well, has been largely overlooked. After nearly 40 years of counseling and more than 25 years on the staff of the Johns Hopkins Comprehensive Diabetes Center, I have seen that the best managers of diabetes are both diabetes smart and stress smart. To successfully manage diabetes, stress needs to be contained, avoided when possible, and kept to a minimum when unavoidable.

Even though you may have the strong support of family and friends and the guidance of healthcare providers, the ultimate responsibility for managing the disease is yours. Diabetes care is 95–99% self-care. You are the one who lives with diabetes day by day, hour by hour. You are the one who is continually making decisions regarding glucose management. In most instances, you are the only one who can contain the stress of diabetes and other stress producers in your life.

You probably have found diabetes stressful at least some of the time; you may find it distressing a lot of the time. In addition, you may be coping with some of the many everyday sources of stress. Excessive stress—extreme in intensity and/or duration—can seriously complicate diabetes management. The following fascinating study illustrates how stress can affect blood glucose levels.

A native Italian with type 1 diabetes was monitored continually using a glucose sensor attached to his skin. On the first day, his blood glucose level varied from 105 to 150 mg/dL. The next day, his activities were very similar to those of the first day, with one exception: he went to watch his favorite soccer team play a match. Once the game started, his blood glucose level began to rise. At a critical point in the game, the level peaked at 302 mg/dL. He had not eaten for several hours. The dramatic rise in his blood glucose level was a reaction to stress.

Europeans tend to be fanatical about their soccer. The subject of this study saw the possibility of his team losing, and he perceived this as a threat, which triggered the stress response. The result was a considerable increase in his blood glucose level. The stress response, often referred to as the fight-or-flight response, is a physiological and psychological reaction to the perception of danger. The soccer fan's reaction was comparable to the reaction of the prehistoric caveman who is suddenly confronted by a vicious saber-toothed tiger. Seeing the tiger activates the fight-or-flight response, which causes a range of hormonal activity that prepares the caveman to run or fight the beast. These hormonal changes have immediate effects on body and mind.

The fight-or-flight response is invaluable in the presence of real danger, but there are many situations in modern times for which the response is over-reactive. Concerns about finances or the well-being of a loved one can be serious matters, but mobilizing as if it was a physical threat would be a false alarm. Imagine fire engines responding to a false alarm—high costs with no benefits. Excessive stress may be harmful, sometimes permanently. In addition to raising blood glucose levels, too much stress can increase blood pressure and diminish the effectiveness of the immune system. Anything that feels threatening can trigger the stress response. The fear of complications or concerns about a sudden drop in blood glucose levels could be your saber-toothed tiger.

Fear and other emotions are generally a reaction to what is believed to be happening in a given situation. Everyone is a product of his or her beliefs. We perceive danger when we believe that there is danger. Whether the situation is dangerous or not, the result is the same—mind and body respond in a dramatic way. The stress response is described in detail in Chapters 1 and 2. Unfortunately, there are aspects of diabetes, and of modern times in general, that tend to arouse the perception of danger or the intensification of a serious situation. The successful stress manager distinguishes between beliefs that are real and those that are based on assumptions, myths, and other mistruths. Making this distinction is a central theme for this book.

Goals

This book has four major goals:

- To encourage you to make the control of stress a high priority by raising your awareness of the symptoms and effects of excessive stress.
- To provide the best tools and mindset for controlling the stress of diabetes and of life in general.
- To inform you of the value, power, and ways of a mindful approach to managing the stress of diabetes and of life in general.
- To provide you with the power of mindfulness and the competence to live mindfully and thus maximize your overall well-being.

You will learn everything you need to know to manage the stress in your life, a goal that everyone with diabetes should pursue. In fact, it is a goal everyone should pursue.

Stress is not always undesirable; sometimes tension and anxiety are helpful. Stress can motivate us to do something we should do but wouldn't do without the pressure to do it. Would you stick yourself three or four times a day if you didn't have serious concerns about managing your diabetes? To manage diabetes well, it is essential to avoid unnecessary or excessive stress when possible and to minimize the effects of stress when it is unavoidable.

Organization

This book is divided into five sections: Part 1, the basics of stress; Part 2, a foundation for managing stress; Part 3, the tools for containing stress; Part 4, a view of the challenges of raising a child with type 1 diabetes; and Part 5, some final reflections on the power of a mindful approach to stress and diabetes management. Part 5 also provides numerous resources to explore in print and on the Internet related to the material presented in this book.

PART 1

Part 1 covers the basics of stress: what it is and what it does. You will learn what causes stress and how to gauge your stress level. Chapter 1 describes in detail the interactions between stress, the body, and diabetes. Chapter 2 is about the effects of stress on the mind and the subsequent impact on diabetes management. With these chapters, you will understand how stress complicates the managing of diabetes and how it can be a hazard to your health in general.

PART 2

Part 2 presents the infrastructure—the foundation for success-fully managing stress. Chapter 3 introduces the concept of living mindfully. Being mindful (i.e., being aware of what is going on, of what you are thinking and feeling, and of the range of choices in each situation) is fundamental to all of the skills and techniques in this book. If you are living mindlessly—operating on automatic pilot, acting habitually, and not being aware of the choices and possibilities that you have when challenged—then you are experiencing a lot of unnecessary stress. A primary goal here is to help you make the shift from living mindlessly to living mindfully and to achieving the optimum state of personal empowerment—optimum levels of competence and confidence.

If you were about to undertake an important and challenging journey, a venture that might entail some risk to your well-being, what would you do before getting underway? Hopefully, you would prepare by gathering all of the resources you will need for success. You would mindfully plan and prepare to succeed. Managing diabetes is a lifelong journey that can be seriously challenged by stress. Having a mindful approach that uses a range of skills for avoiding or minimizing potential stressors is putting yourself in the best possible place for a successful journey.

Mindful questions throughout this book will guide you in developing a mindful way of thinking and living, which is essential for controlling stress and managing diabetes. Questioning what is happening and why and determining what choices you have prevents the tendency to act and react automatically or, worse, impulsively. Asking the right questions is essential to arriving at the right answers.

In *Man Is Not Alone: A Philosophy of Religion* (2), the eminent scholar and theologian Abraham J. Heschel wrote, "The question is the beginning of all thinking. In knowing how to ask the right question lies the only hope of arriving at an answer." A primary purpose of *The Mindful Guide to Managing Diabetes* is to guide the reader to the right question for any situation that might be faced. The *mindful questions* to apply in a given situation are designated by this symbol:

MQ

In Chapter 4, you will learn the value of setting goals and how to set goals in a meaningful way. At the Johns Hopkins Comprehensive Diabetes Center's educational programs, patients made a contract to achieve a goal. The specific behavior changes necessary for accomplishing the goal are included in the written pact. Making a contract for yourself is making a commitment, a vow to pursue a self-determined goal. Setting a goal, putting it in written form, and planning to achieve it maximizes the probability of getting where you want to be. Each of these steps is presented in this chapter.

Diabetes arouses feelings that can be a major source of stress. In fact, the relationship between stress and emotions is cyclical. A feeling can cause stress that, in turn, intensifies the emotion and vice versa. Furthermore, stress can bring on a feeling that worsens the initial stress. Although our tendency is to avoid unpleasant feelings (the sale of drugs to suppress discomforting feelings is a multi-billion dollar business), you will learn in Chapter 5 how to make good use of feelings of sadness, anxiety, fear, and anger. You will learn how to use these unpleasant feelings to respond adaptively rather than to react impulsively or possibly destructively. If you accidentally put your hand on a hot stove, the pain is a vital signal to remove your hand before any more damage is done to it. In the same way, uncomfortable feelings can be a valuable signal to mindfully choose an appropriate response to whatever is causing the discomfort. Emotional control is not about eliminating negative feelings; it is about being emotionally smart and thereby recognizing and responding to these emotions effectively.

For many individuals, interactions with other people are a primary source of stress. Perhaps you have someone in your life who is a member of the diabetes police, someone who continually tells you what to do or not do to manage your diabetes. Chapter 6 offers three essential people skills—communicating effectively, being assertive, and resolving conflicts—for dealing effectively with others in a variety of situations and thus preventing unnecessary strife.

Maintaining a positive and invigorating lifestyle will prevent a great deal of unnecessary and unwanted stress. Eating healthfully and exercising regularly are essential to a healthy lifestyle. Chapter 7 covers aspects of lifestyle that are not usually included in books and educational programs, including the roles of creativity, gratitude, and support in having a healthy and productive life. You will learn how maintaining a balance of work, play, and rest is important and that fatigue caused by lack of sleep or by an overly heavy work schedule can often be eased by some healthy fun.

PART 3

Part 3 is your toolbox. These chapters provide a range of tools for containing the stress of diabetes or any other stressor in your life. Each chapter covers a technique for preventing stress and/or keeping unavoidable stress to a minimum.

Reframing, the subject of Chapter 8, is one of the most powerful tools for managing stress. Each of us is a product of our beliefs. Some of us are victims of a belief system that is distorted or misdirected. With mindful awareness, you can recognize frames (beliefs) that are not working for you and replace them with frames that have positive consequences. It is taking charge of your belief system, the engine that drives your thoughts, feelings, and behavior. A central theme throughout the book is that choice is power, and reframing—changing a faulty belief to a sound and useful one—is always a choice.

The frame of letting go is relevant to many stressful situations. Chapter 9 is devoted to the option of freeing yourself from something stressful as opposed to holding on to it, even though the stressor is causing you considerable agony. Holding on to faulty beliefs that result in maladaptive patterns and habits is acting mindlessly; giving up these unfavorable patterns and habits is gaining significant control of your life.

Chapter 10 presents a playbook of frames divided into two categories: sure winners and sure losers. The frames of "maybe," "gratitude," and "fascination" are powerful stress-busters included in the chapter. In contrast, the frames of "perfection" and "denial" and ones that are based on "should," "must," or "never" are examples of sure stress-builders.

There are times when we may believe that life is just one problem after another. Certainly, managing diabetes is managing a variety of problems—often, seemingly, one after another. Being good at problem solving is an essential aspect of stress control. Chapter 11 presents a step-by-step approach to solving problems. Because your strengths will play an important role in solving many kinds of problems, you will learn how to identify your strengths and make them stronger.

Anticipating a potential problem can be the easiest way to avoid unnecessary stress. Chapter 12 reviews specific scenarios that people with diabetes commonly experience with consistently negative results. Suppose, for example, that you are going to visit family on a holiday and you know that they cook and eat in ways that do not suit you. What can you do to avoid an unpleasant outcome? When you anticipate the problem, you have time to take the steps necessary to take care of yourself.

The benefits of humor, mirth, and laughter are the focus of Chapter 13. Research has shown that creating moments of fun and happiness have positive results in relieving physical and mental suffering. Hospitals and cancer centers around the country use audiovisual recordings to provide patients the opportunity to get some respite from their pain and anxiety. The saying "laughter is the best medicine" has proven to have merit for many individuals who are dealing with illness or another hardship . . . if only briefly.

In Chapter 14, the Internet is explored for its value as a resource for information and assistance in managing both stress and diabetes. Various aspects of the Internet and the World Wide Web are profiled from several angles: what they offer, how to use them, and their potential benefits and evils. Websites, apps, podcasts, portals, and text messaging are scrutinized in the context of managing diabetes and stress.

Diabetes-specific apps provide a variety of services for improving the user's ability to manage the disease: continuous monitoring and tracking of self-management tasks, sending self-management tips, and delivering clinically accurate feedback when needed. There are apps that accept real-time patient data and provide patients with direct feedback from healthcare professionals or from automated systems. Some apps provide the means to chat with others who have diabetes. With the vast availability of mobile phones, these services are accessible in rural areas of the United States and in developing countries worldwide, areas that would otherwise have very limited access to valuable information regarding diabetes care. Whether or not the information and services provided by an app or website are valid is evaluated in this segment.

Meditation, the subject of Chapter 15, is an effective and versatile stress-buster, efficient both in rapidly reducing stress and in developing a resistance to becoming stressed. Specific instructions for several types of meditation are described in detail: a basic breathing technique, variations of the basic method, and a diabetes-specific method.

A vital addition to Chapter 15 is the introduction of mindful meditation. *Mindfulness* is a way of living, a state of mind that optimizes one's awareness, decision-making, self-control, and self-esteem. It is the core of the approach to controlling stress presented throughout this book. *Mindful meditation* is an act of deliberate contemplation. In addition to achieving the numerous benefits of meditation per se, practice develops and reinforces a mindful approach to everyday life.

PART 4

Part 4 focuses on dealing with the numerous stressors associated with type 1 diabetes. The causes of type 1 and type 2 diabetes are different. For type 1 diabetes, the immune system mistakenly attacks and demolishes the body's healthy β-cells as though they are a harmful foreign body. Without the insulin-producing β-cells, the pancreas is unable to produce insulin, which is essential for regulating blood glucose levels. Consequently, people with type 1 diabetes use injections of insulin to replace what the body is no longer capable of producing. Type 1 diabetes usually develops in childhood or adolescence. However, although relatively rare, this form of the disease can develop later in life.

People with type 2 diabetes produce insulin, but the body is unable to use it effectively. With the body resisting the insulin, the pancreas tries to overcome the problem by producing more of this vital hormone, causing a dangerous accumulation in the bloodstream. This form of diabetes can develop in preadolescence, and the rate of occurrence increases substantially with aging. The 2017 National Diabetes Statistics Report noted that there are 30.3 million people in the U.S. with diabetes, of which 90–95% have type 2 diabetes.

Chapter 16: Stress and Type 1 Diabetes is about having a mindful approach to raising a child with type 1 diabetes. For the parents or another primary caregiver, the sources of stress are numerous. A range of stressors is included: the strain and tension that originates within a parent, from the child, or from siblings and others. Given that stress can impede the ability to effectively meet the numerous challenges imposed in raising the youngster, addressing these demands mindfully maximizes one's ability to remain calm, to think clearly, and to make the right decisions when under pressure.

PART 5

The Afterword, in Part 5, offers my final reflections on the principles set forth in this book:

- Stress control is essential for managing diabetes well.
- Living mindfully is empowering for all aspects of a healthy life.
- The essence of our thoughts, feelings, and actions is what we believe in the moment.
- Living mindfully gives one the opportunity to "reframe" a faulty, potentially harmful, belief.

As you learn from reading this book, you will know that in every moment there are choices and possibilities for you to not only take good care of yourself but to also significantly enrich the quality of your life. By claiming the powers of the mindful approach, you can minimize the stress in your life and maintain good diabetes management.

A final segment, Resources, includes References (a list of writings relevant to the subject of this work) and a list of Suggested Readings (a collection of books that may not be diabetes-specific but are pertinent to living well with the disease). And, as a complement to Chapter 14 (The Internet: Excellent with Caution), there is an index of well-regarded websites, apps, and podcasts to enhance your self-care capability.

PART 1

Connecting the Dots: Stress and Diabetes

CHAPTER 1

Stress, Your Body, and Diabetes

Stress is a commanding subject in today's society. You hear it mentioned frequently in conversation with friends and loved ones. When you read your daily newspaper, watch the news on television, or peruse the self-help section in a library or bookstore, you are offered a variety of solutions to relieve day-to-day stress. The reality is that we have many potential stressors in our daily lives; we have personal concerns at work or home, and we have anxiety about the economy, the environment, the cost of medical care, the prevalence of crime, and hateful biases. Early life adversities and various negative personal traits such as tendencies toward denial, aggression, or hostility are known causes of stress and its harmful consequences. Or perhaps it is your children and/or parents who are the source of anxiety and strife.

An annual survey by the American Psychological Association (Stress in America: The State of Our Nation, 2017) reported that three of four Americans experienced at least one stress symptom in the last month. A total of 45% reported lying awake at night, 36% reported feeling nervous or anxious, 35% reported irritability or anger, and 34% reported fatigue due to stress. In an annual Gallup survey (2018), a majority of Americans (55%) said they had experienced stress during a lot of the day and nearly half (45%) said they felt worried a lot. This placed the United States in seventh place among the 10 most stressed populations in the world that ranged from 52 to 59 percent. The World Health Organization has stated that stress has become a "worldwide epidemic."

An addiction to mobile devices has resulted in an increasing number of individuals (especially youths) not getting an adequate amount of sleep, resulting in a disturbed circadian rhythm, which combined can cause considerable stress. Not having adequate time to fulfill essential tasks is a common cause of stress. A total of 54% of Americans who do not have enough time to attend to important matters report that they frequently experience stress.

The constant and numerous demands of diabetes add even more stress for someone with the disease. Here is a range of stressors that can affect someone with diabetes:

- The vigilance and discipline that diabetes management demands.
- Feeling deprived of favorite foods.
- Feeling inferior for having diabetes.
- A sense of isolation from family.
- A sense of loss.
- Fear of developing a complication.
- Having a complication.
- When necessities of life conflict with the necessities of diabetes care.
- The financial cost of diabetes care.
- Lack of understanding and support.
- Being overly dependent on others.
- Excessive, unwarranted pressure from others.
- Blood glucose level not consistent with effort being made for good diabetes management.
- Fear of severe hypoglycemia.
- Fear of having to use insulin.
- Dealing with the need to make well-established lifestyle changes (such as changing eating habits or stopping smoking).
- Lack of adequate medical services.
- Lack of knowledge about diabetes care.

Any of these issues can be a serious deterrent to successful diabetes management. Excessive or extreme stress is a grave threat to one's health and general well-being. The focus throughout this book will be on keeping the level of stress as low as possible by avoiding, eliminating, or moderating the stressors of diabetes and life in general. But, before presenting the means of controlling these stressors, let's look at what stress is and what impact it has on your health. In this chapter, the effects of stress on the body are addressed. In Chapter 2, the effects on the mind are explored. Stress is not "just" something that is uncomfortable; it can, in fact, cause significant damage to your body, including affecting your diabetes both directly and indirectly.

What Is Stress?

Stress is a reaction to a perceived threat. The reaction is generally both physical and emotional and can be very intense, regardless of whether the threat is real or imagined. You may have heard this reaction referred to as the "fight-or-flight response." This designation refers to the survival aspect of the stress response; it prepares the body and mind to cope with the threat—to fight or flee from danger.

Not all stress is unhealthy. When the intensity of the response is consistent with the intensity of the threat, the stress response is appropriate, if not essential. For example, complications are a threat to most people with diabetes. Some degree of stress is likely to motivate you to do what is necessary to manage the disease to minimize the dreaded risk of complications. If you didn't have some fear of complications or of some other troubling aspect of diabetes, what would entice you to stick yourself to draw blood several times a day or to resist eating something that you know will be so yummy? Your concerns about the consequences of doing or not doing something motivate healthy behavior, even when it is difficult to do. Stress in daily life that is an appropriate response to the situation is termed eustress (good stress). A reasonable degree of tension and uneasiness is expected in anticipation of getting married, being promoted at work, or moving far from home. If, however, the stress is not managed well, it will have a detrimental impact on what would otherwise be a normal experience.

The occurrence of stress is complicated by the fact that—depending on the way your nervous system has been programmed—your perception of a threat can be unreal or exaggerated. Consequently, the stress response can be unwarranted, a false alarm, or overly intense. In addition, although the nervous system is designed to respond adaptively to stress, it can become overwhelmed by the chronic stress that is so common in modern times. Persistent, uncontrolled stress is harmful to the immune system and to health in general.

Unfortunately, there are many things in life that can trigger the stress response. Inappropriate, overly intense, or prolonged stress responses can result in a range of undesirable consequences. For the individual with diabetes, the results can be even more troublesome. Excessive stress generally increases blood glucose levels, complicates glycemic management, and makes taking care of oneself more difficult.

What Does the Fight-or-Flight Response Do?

Put yourself in the situation of a caveman who has just come face-to-face with a mean-looking saber-toothed tiger. You quickly try to decide how best to survive this situation—do you run and hopefully escape the beast, or do you fight it? Either way, you will need a body that is equipped to handle the situation—and fast!

In this or any other situation that is perceived as a threat, as soon as your brain recognizes danger, it releases an array of stress hormones, including adrenaline, cortisol, epinephrine, and norepinephrine. They, in turn, activate the systems needed to survive this threat, causing them to pump up to their maximum levels. All activities not needed to fight or run are reduced or minimized. The message of the fight-or-flight response is to prepare the body to be as fast, strong, and invulnerable as possible. As a result, numerous changes take place in the body:

- Eyes dilate to see better.
- Cardiovascular output increases to deliver oxygen and energy to muscles, which means that heart rate and blood pressure increase. (At a very high stress level, heart output may be five times greater than at rest.)
- Major arteries constrict to increase pressure, so blood is delivered with greater speed.
- Blood becomes more viscous to avoid excessive bleeding if injured.
- Breathing increases rapidly to increase oxygen supply.
- Blood flow to the digestive tract decreases to send more blood to the brain and muscles, where it is most needed. In fact, the digestive system pretty much shuts down. (The discomfort of indigestion won't matter if you don't survive the tiger.)
- Blood flow to the muscles in the arms and legs increases.
- The body's sense of pain is dulled.
- Immune system function diminishes. (After all, fighting infection is secondary to surviving the jaws of a tiger.)
- The reproductive system slows down. Menstrual cycles can become irregular or stop; sperm count and testosterone levels may decline, which *might* help explain the problem of trying to have a baby when the wish to conceive is stressful.
- The kidneys conserve water by reabsorbing it into the circulatory system, which causes wear and tear on the kidneys. (In fight-or-flight mode, hydration is essential, but there is no time to stop and have a nice beverage.)
- **The liver produces glucose to power the muscles and brain, raising the blood glucose level.**
- **As the level of glucose increases, more insulin is needed for the glucose to be used by the body cells for energy, which can be troublesome in a person with diabetes.**

Each of the changes imposed by the fight-or-flight response can have undesirable consequences. The last two changes (in bold type)—an increase in glucose and an increase in demand for insulin—are of special concern with regard to managing blood glucose levels.

Stress—real or imagined—can pose serious health problems for anyone, with or without diabetes. The causes of stress can be physical, such as an illness, surgery, or injury from an accident. Even having a cold or flu can hamper glucose management. Many stressors are mental, like concerns about work, family, the economy, and crime. Whether the stress is physical or mental, both the body and the mind are affected.

With diabetes, there are the relentless demands that add both physical and emotional stress to the mix. Think about the stress you sometimes feel as a result of managing your diabetes day to day. Do you worry about developing complications, having an excessively low blood glucose level, or having to start using insulin? Does the daily regimen of checking blood glucose levels and the vigilance and discipline required to manage diabetes wear you down?

Remember that each time one of these concerns provokes anxiety or anger, your heart, blood vessels, kidneys, digestive and immune systems, and blood glucose level are prompted to act. The cumulative effects of these disturbances can cause or worsen an illness as well as impede effective diabetes management.

The stress response was adaptive for the caveman threatened by a hungry tiger. If he survived the beast, his body systems returned to normal. But there are numerous ways in which the fight-or-flight response can be activated in modern times—over and over again and sometimes continually. Remember the Italian man whose blood glucose level soared to 302 mg/dL while he was watching a soccer match? The possibility that his favorite team might lose the match was so alarming to him that it initiated the fight-or-flight response. The brain has not caught up with modern times; it tends to perceive far too many saber-toothed tigers. The stress response was intended to protect us from physical harm, but it also reacts to psychological threats—real or not—which can be just as troubling, if not more so.

DOES STRESS AFFECT YOUR GLUCOSE LEVEL?

With diabetes, mental or emotional stress is likely to increase your blood glucose levels. Here is a simple procedure that gives you a sense of the effect of stress on your glucose level:

- Step 1: Before you check your blood glucose level, evaluate your mental stress level on a scale of 1 to 10 (with 10 being the highest possible and 0 being no stress at all). Write this number down.
- Step 2: Check your blood glucose level, and write it down next to the stress evaluation.
- Step 3: Track these numbers for a week or more. At the end of the period, look for a pattern. You may want to try graphing the numbers to visually spot any trends.

Answer these *mindful questions*:

MQ | *Are your blood glucose levels higher when your estimated stress levels are high?*

Are your blood glucose levels lower when your stress levels are low?

If you answer "yes" to either question, then mental stress is probably influencing your blood glucose management. Keep in mind that other factors may be in effect. However, if there is a consistent connection over a few weeks, it's reasonable to conclude that there is a relationship between your stress level and blood glucose level.

In fact, anything viewed as a threat can activate the stress response. The demands of diabetes add to the risk of such events occurring too often without the benefit of the break that the caveman had between battles. Although stress presents immediate problems, chronic stress can have even more serious results.

What Are the Effects of Chronic Stress?

Stress can affect your blood glucose level both directly and indirectly. A change in blood glucose level can occur immediately when the fight-or-flight response is activated. A perceived threat triggers the release of stress hormones, which, in turn, tends to raise blood glucose levels regardless of whether food has been eaten recently. More specifically, release of the hormone cortisol stimulates the liver to secrete glucose into the blood and converts stored fat cells into usable fuel. These changes provide the body with extra energy via an increase in glucose to the body's cells. Furthermore, with the increase in glucose, there is a need for more insulin to ensure that the glucose is converted into usable energy by muscle cells.

However, if you have type 2 diabetes, your pancreas may not be able to produce enough insulin, or there may be a problem with using the insulin that is secreted. If the cells are not able to use the additional glucose, then it builds up in the blood. If the stress is long term, there is the possibility of a dangerous buildup of blood glucose levels, possibly leading to ketoacidosis.

Research has shown that the effect of stress on blood glucose levels in people with diabetes may be even more complicated. It may depend on the type of diabetes you have and whether the stress is physical or mental. For people with type 1 diabetes, the impact of mental stress—such as a job change or an assignment deadline—on glucose levels has been mixed. For some individuals, blood glucose levels actually go down with mental stress; others are likely to have an increase. People with type 2 diabetes, though, tend to have an increase in blood glucose levels as a result of mental stress. In the face of physical stress, individuals with type 1 or type 2 diabetes tend to show raised blood glucose levels. Refer to the text on page 21 to find a simple way to determine whether stress may be affecting your blood glucose levels.

Researchers have found that decreasing stress may have a different direct impact on blood glucose levels for people with type 1 or type 2 diabetes. If you have type 1 diabetes, you may not see an immediate reduction in your glucose level after reducing mental stress. Regardless of the type of diabetes, decreasing your stress will have a positive impact on your over-all control by eliminating barriers to successful self-care. Stress is a drain on energy and a distraction from what needs to be done. Eliminating it increases energy and the ability to think and act more effectively.

Stress affects blood glucose levels indirectly by having a negative impact on self-care. When you feel stressed out, you may not take good care of yourself because you are distracted by tension and anxiety. Reacting to the demands of diabetes with anger is another serious deterrent to exercising good self-care. The lack of focus may lead to making unhealthy choices, such as not exercising, drinking too much alcohol, or not checking blood glucose levels. Perhaps of most impor-tance to someone with diabetes is the risk of overeating in an attempt to soothe the discomfort of feeling distressed. Rich foods can be very gratifying in the short run; however, using food and drink for emotional comfort can have devastating consequences over time.

Chronic stress is very hard on the heart and vascular network of veins and arteries. In the fight-or-flight mode, the heart is pumping harder and faster to get blood to the muscles as quickly as possible. The increase in blood pressure is an unwelcome consequence for people who already have high blood pressure. Furthermore, blood vessels have to contract to create the pres-sure needed for faster movement of the blood and to decrease the flow to parts of the body not involved in mobilizing to run or fight. The increase in the force of the blood on the vessels causes significant wear and tear over time. If there is already damage in the vessels, the wear and tear will likely be more troublesome. Because individuals with diabetes have a high incidence of coronary disease, avoiding the effects of stress on the heart and vascular system is important.

The body also increases the amount of fats in the bloodstream to provide more energy during the fight-or-flight response. However, just as with glucose, the body may not be able to metabolize frequent, unnecessary secretions of extra fats due to stress. These extra fats then remain in your bloodstream and may contribute to the buildup of plaque in the blood vessels. Such plaque buildup can result in a heart attack or stroke. Furthermore, when faced with a modern-day equivalent of the saber-toothed tiger, the blood thickens to restrict bleeding in the event of being wounded. For individuals who are dealing with obstructions in the blood vessels, thickened blood presents a greater risk of a serious coronary event, such as a stroke.

When the excessive fuel in the blood is not used for physical activities and more stress hormones accumulate, the risk of serious consequences increases. Some of the potential problems include damage to the immune system, digestive disorders, short-term memory loss, premature coronary artery disease, and even a heart attack.

The stress response can impair immune function, which increases vulnerability to other illnesses. In fact, research indicates that prolonged stress can permanently damage the immune system. The fight-or-flight response also decreases the blood flow to the digestive tract. This change leaves mucous linings vulnerable to acids, which can cause ulcers to develop. An ulcer can lead to further food restrictions and physical discomfort. Furthermore, prolonged stress worsens fatigue and causes digestive disorders and impotence. It also can damage eyes, kidneys, and the brain. The impact of chronic stress on thoughts and feelings is described in Chapter 2.

Am I Stressed Out?

When you learn to recognize the core symptoms of stress, you will be able to manage stress more successfully. The following conditions are some of the most common ways in which stress is experienced.

- Sleeping too much or not enough
- Fatigue
- Changes in appetite (eating more or less)
- Significant weight loss or gain
- Crying frequently
- Trouble with memory and/or concentration
- Anxious thoughts (often taking the form of "what if . . .")
- Muscle tension (that crick in your neck)
- Feeling irritable, uneasy, or on edge
- Symptoms of depression (see Chapter 2)
- Stomach problems (vomiting, nausea, stomachaches, diarrhea, constipation)
- Loss of interest in sex
- Avoiding work or school tasks and/or difficulty completing them
- General lack of motivation
- Changes in relationships (either avoiding or feeling the need to seek out the company of others more than usual)
- Headaches
- Feeling your heart beating (often occurs when trying to fall asleep)
- Difficulty swallowing or feeling as though you are choking
- Trembling, shakiness
- Feeling faint
- Sweating profusely
- Grinding your teeth

As you probably are aware, some of the symptoms on the list are common to hypoglycemia and hyperglycemia, so it is important to take that into consideration. However, when you experience one or more of these symptoms, consider the possibility that the discomfort is stress related, especially when your blood glucose level is not extremely low or high. If it is stress, the challenge is to identify its cause. The *mindful questions* are:

MQ | *What is causing me to feel stressed? Is it a faulty belief or frame?*
|
| *When did the discomfort start and what was going on at that time?*

Other *mindful questions* may arise from these basic ones:

MQ | *Did I start having these tension headaches after my boss turned down my raise?*
|
| *When did I start having trouble sleeping and what was going on at that time?*
|
| *Did anything happen that is upsetting me and causing this discomfort?*
|
| *Why did my stomach start hurting a few days ago?*

It will be helpful to keep track of your stress symptoms. Most of us seem to be partial to certain ways of experiencing our stress. Being mindful of the symptoms that are common for you is an important step in managing stress. The more aware you are of being stressed, the better able you will be to understand what is causing it, which is essential for minimizing the strain. As you progress through this book, you will understand how awareness at every level of thinking and feeling will serve you well in managing both stress and diabetes.

Summing Up the Impact of Stress

We know that the fight-or-flight response is important in the face of true danger; it initiates changes in the body that maximize the chance of survival. However, when the situation is falsely perceived as a threat, the body will mobilize to fight or take flight. Real or imagined, the stress response can seriously impair the ability to manage your diabetes, especially when the stress is prolonged and excessive. Furthermore, too much stress can cause other serious medical problems. These possible consequences are especially important because the demands of diabetes tend to be stressful for so many who have it. The demands of trying to manage diabetes can be stressful; the stress, in turn, makes the management of diabetes even more challenging. This troubling cycle emphasizes the value of being a world-class stress manager.

The following message is important: a key to managing your diabetes is managing your stress. It is important to be mindful of when you are becoming stressed out and to address the situation to prevent a continuation of the stress response. To this end, you will want to increase your awareness of patterns of stress and work toward avoiding potential stressors or keeping the impact of a stressful situation at a minimum. Learning the signs and symptoms of being stressed out will be an invaluable aid in alerting you when there is a stress-producing problem to fix. Being aware of the presence of stress gives you the opportunity to use any of the skills and strategies you will learn throughout this book. However, if you think you are experiencing stress-related increases in glucose, consult with your doctor, since adjustments to medications may be needed.

The focus of this chapter has been on the effects of stress on the body and on the management of diabetes. In the next chapter, the focus is on the mental and emotional effects of stress and how these effects can cause behavior that is counterproductive to good self-care.

CHAPTER 2

Stress, Your Mind, and Diabetes

The ways that stress affects the body and glucose management were addressed in Chapter 1. Here, the focus is on how stress can affect the quality of your life. Stress can determine how you think, feel, and behave; it can play havoc with the ability to manage diabetes. Understand that although these chapters treat the body and mind separately, in reality, these are not disconnected entities. It is practical to consider them separately, but not recognizing their intricate, immediate, and interactive connection is a mistake. The reality is that if you disturb the body, you disturb the mind and vice versa. That this fact has not been fully recognized and accepted in general medicine has been a serious problem in diagnosing and treating many suffering individuals.

How Does Stress Affect the Mind?

THINKING AND STRESS

Stress is to thinking as lightening and static are to television reception. It is disruptive, distracting, and dysfunctional.

The successful management of diabetes requires a lot of thinking. The management of diabetes can be described as a process of almost continual decision making and problem solving. "I am going to eat soon. Is there something I have to do now?" "I just ate more than I intended. What should I do?" "This game of tennis has been longer and harder than I expected.

What do I have to do to cover for it?" "I am feeling a bit shaky. Should I check my blood or just eat something that will raise my blood glucose level?" The problem is that stress affects the ability to think clearly, which impairs the ability to make sound decisions and solve problems effectively.

A preoccupation with unpleasant concerns or fears makes it difficult, if not impossible, to concentrate on a task or an objective. Remember that a perceived threat signals mind and body to prepare for danger. The distraction is formidable. Furthermore, persistent worry impairs memory, which is already idiosyncratic—we don't always remember events the way they actually happened. The situation is similar to an overloaded electrical circuit; where there is too much to deal with, it shuts down. With too much to think about, thought processes are disrupted and cognitive functioning suffers. To make matters worse, thoughts use energy even when they are not acted upon. Thus, a relentless stream of thoughts can be exhausting and add to the stress already occurring.

FEELINGS AND STRESS

Stress activates intense emotions that may overwhelm rational thinking. Have you ever been so frustrated with managing your glucose levels that you wanted to give up?

Given that stress is a reaction to a perceived danger, feelings are a natural and intense part of the stress response. Anger, fear, and sadness are common reactions to a threat. Although these emotions may be appropriate and even essential in the face of real danger, they can be counterproductive when the risk of harm is not real or is greatly exaggerated. Being preoccupied with feelings of anger or fear is not helpful when you are confronted with a problem that needs thoughtful consideration and sound decision making.

But it could be even worse. The survival mode—an ancient reflexive system—is the default mode in the face of danger. Humans are wired, first and foremost, to survive. The system for rational, objective thinking is relatively new in the development of the brain and nervous system. Consequently, we are configured to respond emotionally before thinking rationally about what is going on. Imagine that you are about to take your diabetes medication when you receive word that you did not get the job you had applied for. The combination of sadness, frustration, and, perhaps, fear and anger could totally distract you from taking the medication. Hopefully, you will think about taking the medication in a reasonable time.

The daily news provides stories of individuals who have impulsively acted upon their feelings and have done stupid or vicious things. Negative emotions can be both a prevalent and powerful source of stress and a debilitating consequence of stress. A comprehensive discussion of the need to be emotionally smart is provided in Chapter 5.

Have you ever said, "I'm worried to death about . . ." or "I'm so worried over . . ."? Perhaps, the correct question should have been, "How often do you make such downbeat, distressing remarks?" Worrying is inevitable, and it can be very stressful. Family and others have heard me say, "There's only one reason to have children, and that is to have something to worry about for the rest of your life . . . and then you have grandchildren."

When we worry continually in anticipation of an event or a situation that will occur in the future, the degree of anxiety will increase as the dreaded happening approaches. Growing up with a faulty belief—"I am a loser and I will fail at anything I try"—can be a lifelong source of stress. And as noted in the previous chapter, the uncertainty of change, even when it is a positive transformation, can cause a prolonged state of worry and anguish. People who are prone to anxiety have difficulty unburdening themselves of worry.

BEHAVIOR AND STRESS

The diminished thinking and intense feelings that come with stress can fuel self-defeating behavior. Under the weight of stress, sound thinking is disrupted, and imposing feelings can push or pull you one way or another. Chances are that the results of your stress-induced behavior will suffer. Although there are situations for which the right behavior is obvious and requires little, if any, thinking, the most vital situations need careful thought, often in the face of intense feelings. The conditions imposed by the fight-or-flight response are the opposite of the conditions needed to react effectively to complex or challenging circumstances.

Imagine that you learned that a dear friend had said that it disturbed her when you checked your blood glucose. The message triggered strong feelings of sadness and anger, and you immediately text to inform her of how disappointed you are and that you will spare her further discomfort by staying away from her. Obviously, those feelings have impaired your ability to think clearly. First, you did not hear the remark directly so you cannot be certain that your dear friend said what you were told. Second, if she did make that remark, would it not be better to have a conversation with her about it? Would it be helpful to know exactly what bothered her? The impulsive behavior was driven by feelings of resentment and would be counterproductive.

Think of yourself as a train moving forward with the intent to continue going straight as it approaches a railroad switch. But as the train comes to the switch, the rails move and you are suddenly going in a direction you did not expect or choose. Similarly, in the scenario described above, you are doing your thing until you are told that a friend was upset when you checked your blood glucose. Whether you felt belittled or, perhaps, betrayed, you mindlessly switched to a hostile manner. Now, seeing your friend as a threat (the historic saber-toothed tiger), you automatically went into stress mode. If we don't learn how to control our emotions, they will determine our behavior. The mindful approach presented throughout this book will give you that control.

How Does Mental Stress Affect Diabetes Management?

The challenge for someone with diabetes often occurs when there is a conflict between two choices: choosing between French fries and a vegetable is a simple, but pertinent, example. To resist the temptation to go for the fries requires clear, calm thinking—a state of mind that is jeopardized when feeling stressed.

> *Alex's blood glucose level is dropping, and he is feeling jittery. The problem is that he has a deadline to meet, and he is determined to finish the project as quickly as possible. He believes that he has to finish it "no matter what." Alex is mentally stressed, and the pressure imposed by his view of the deadline has blinded Alex to any other choice and to the probable consequences of his behavior. The fear of not meeting the deadline overwhelms good judgment.*

To deal with the situation effectively, Alex will have to pause and reflect on what is happening. He will need to recognize that he is being driven by feelings that are, in turn, being fueled by the belief that delaying the completion of the project will have serious, negative consequences. In the next chapter, you will learn the means of asking **mindful questions** to prevent or minimize stress. The **mindful questions** for Alex's problem are:

MQ | *Will the brief time it takes to check my blood glucose and ingest something that raises my blood glucose level really cause me to miss the deadline?*

In the unlikely event that I miss the deadline, will it really have such dire consequences?

Since I am reasonably sure my glucose level is low, what is the risk of having something to raise the level without taking the time to check?

Is the reward for meeting the deadline worth the risk of having a serious hypoglycemic experience?

Unfortunately, Alex was overtaken by self-imposed stress, and he was losing control of his diabetes.

Poor eating habits may also coincide with having too much stress in one's life. A common cause of obesity is referred to as "emotional eating": eating to soothe unpleasant feelings and relieve tension. Food is used by many to soothe emotional pain. And food is so easy to find! To make matters worse, the foods that are the most soothing tend to be the richest—the more fatty and sugary, the better. Eating may provide some immediate relief from an unpleasant stress-related feeling, but it quickly becomes an obstacle to glycemic management.

In the chapters that follow, you will learn a variety of ways to successfully manage the stressors that are so common to diabetes.

Are There Long-Term Effects of Stress?

Each stressful event takes its toll. Stress consumes an excessive amount of physical and mental energy. It harms the body in the same way as not getting adequate sleep. In addition, the wear and tear of excessive stress diminishes mental functioning.

The effects of too much stress are cyclical. The more stress a person has, the less one is able to deal with it; consequently, the stress level increases. The more stress, the less one is able to properly manage blood glucose levels, which results in more stress.

CAN LONG-TERM STRESS CAUSE DEPRESSION?

Excessive, prolonged stress causes poor glucose levels, which, in turn, leads to frustration and despair or even fear. The next step in this downward emotional spiral is pessimism and resignation, surrendering to defeat. The individual suffering these gloomy feelings begins to believe that managing diabetes is impossible and that the worst is unavoidable. A typical conclusion is, "This is hopeless, so why even try?" These are the unmistakable signs of depression.

When someone is continually besieged by stressful circumstances, the risk of becoming depressed increases. The foundations of depression are feeling hopeless and helpless. These feelings of despair occur when the situation is continually perceived as a threat that is uncontrollable. The perceived threat can be real or imagined; it does not matter. As the threat persists, the reactions become consistent with a state of depression. A state of depression can vary from feeling down or low to being unable to perform basic functions. In addition to being a miserable condition in its own right, any level of depression is a deterrent to the effective management of diabetes and of life in general.

The symptoms of depression—despair, irritability, fatigue, low self-esteem, poor concentration, and a sense of hopelessness and helplessness—work against the positive attitude that is required for managing diabetes. The motivation and ability to take care of oneself and to manage diabetes suffer as a result of being depressed.

Let's look at this connection another way—imagine each stressor as a one-pound weight on your chest. Every day the stressor lasts, it gains another pound. After a period of time, you will feel trapped beneath the weight of all of that stress. If you tried to get up and do anything, it would feel impossible.

Chronic stress creates this feeling in many people. You can see, then, how prolonged, persistent stress could lead to depression. Why bother doing anything when nothing seems to help and nothing seems to change?

The combination of depression and stress increases the risk of other problems. For example, people who are suffering from depression and stress may increase their use of alcohol and other substances or they may smoke more cigarettes. It is not unusual for depression and stress to take a toll on personal relationships—leading to isolation from family and friends. This scenario is a troubling aspect of the interactive, downward spiral of depression and stress because the individual who isolates himself or herself from others is cutting off support that is desperately needed.

Although it is unquestionable that the burden of coping with a serious, chronic disease can lead to becoming depressed, there is a significant risk that people with diabetes can be misdiagnosed with clinical depression. Research indicates that most patients with diabetes and high levels of depressive symptoms are not clinically depressed. The diagnosis of major depression is often based, at least in part, on the results of a rating scale. These studies suggest that the results of these diagnostic instruments are more reflective of diabetes distress than clinical depression. Diabetes distress refers to the unique, often hidden, emotional burdens and worries that are part of the spectrum of patient experience when managing this severe and demanding chronic disease. High levels of diabetes distress have been significantly associated with poor glycemic management, poor self-care, low diabetes self-efficacy, and poor quality of life, even after controlling for clinical depression. High levels of diabetes distress are common and persistent over time, and they are distinct from clinical depression in their linkages with glycemic and disease management. The risk informed by these studies is that patients are being misdiagnosed and, thus, treated ineffectively.

Is There Hope?

As you can see, the impact of stress on the mind is just as important and potentially harmful as its effect on the body. The immediate effects of stress oppose good diabetes management. Chronic stress may lead to debilitating depression, which further diminishes the ability to manage the disease. Unfortunately, there are many ways that diabetes and other conditions can cause and perpetuate a stressful situation. But this is not a hopeless battle.

Studies suggest that stress affects diabetes. While researchers hypothesize that stress may be a factor in the onset of the disease, it is clear that stress can have a harmful impact on glycemic management and on one's general well-being. Recent research, however, indicates that successful stress management can positively improve glycemic management and enhance quality of life. There are straightforward tools that can assist you in managing stress—skills and perspectives that allow better management of diabetes and life in general. By learning how stress can impair your effort to manage diabetes, you have already made progress toward managing essential aspects of life more effectively. This book will assist you in achieving your goal of developing a *mindful* approach that minimizes stress as a deterrent to the optimal management of your diabetes. Each tool will give you a means for living a healthy and content life with diabetes.

PART 2

Back to Basics:
The Fundamentals
of Mastering Stress

CHAPTER 3

Being Mindful

Being mindful is the key to self-control, to the control of stress, to the management of diabetes, and to life in general. Living mindlessly is surrendering control, and it puts you at the risk of chance, impulse, compulsion, the interests of others, and beliefs that may be baseless, if not harmful. The difference between being mindful and being mindless is the difference between being the driver or the passenger on your life journey. It is about taking charge and being in control.

What Does Being Mindful Mean?

Being mindful is paying attention to what you are paying attention to. It is knowing whether you are focused or distracted. It is being in the present, keenly aware of what is happening, both internally and externally. It is being aware of what you are thinking, feeling, and doing, and understanding that your beliefs determine those thoughts, emotions, and actions. Mindfulness is the opposite of living habitually—the opposite of being on automatic pilot. It is the opposite of acting impulsively or compulsively. It is taking command of your life in the most meaningful way possible.

Being mindful is being in the present rather than being distracted by what happened a week ago or years ago or being occupied with what might happen 10 days or 10 months from now. Being in the present does not mean missing the bigger picture. Remembering lessons from the past—good or bad—is essential to successful self-care. But there is a difference between learning from the past and ruminating on it needlessly, especially when the brooding is self-defeating.

The mindful thinker is a keen observer of what is taking place in the moment. When you are mindful, you know what you are thinking and feeling and why. Your observations are objective and, of utmost importance, not judgmental. You react to yourself and the world with wonder and fascination. When your body or emotions sound an alarm, you pay attention.

Have you ever been unkind to someone and at the same time you hear a voice in your head telling you not to act that way? Of course you have. Everyone has had that experience. That voice is your objective observer. Your subjective side—operating on internal processes that disregard reality and yield easily to assumptive thinking and irrational feelings—is the part of you that is being unkind. Living mindfully is being the objective observer. It is being able to get above programmed perceptions, assumptions, and stories that are useless, if not harmful.

A goal of the mindful person is to distinguish right from wrong and fact from fiction. To be mindful is to be weary of denying reality to avoid doing something you don't want to do, especially if it puts you at risk. A mindful person knows the early signs of hypoglycemia, accepts the reality, and acts to prevent a severe drop in blood glucose level. He or she is not distracted from what needs to be done. When you are alert to what is happening and to what choices each situation presents, you are in control. Seeing the range of possibilities greatly reduces stress, and there are almost always a number of choices. Choice is power. Diabetes takes some power away from you, but dealing with it mindlessly will take much more power away than diabetes itself.

When you start paying more attention to what you are thinking about, you may be surprised at how often you are in a mindless state, even though you are indeed thinking. Everyone experiences periods of continuous unedited flow of consciousness, of memories and imaginings. Thinking mindfully is thinking about what you want to think about. It is thinking with reason and purpose. It is sorting out what is fact and what is fiction, and what is real from what may be imagined or believed to be real.

A mindful response is often a creative one. It may require discovering or constructing a different perception of someone or something. If someone is criticizing you for not taking appropriate care of your diabetes, it can be easy to react angrily and lash out at the accuser, creating some stress within and between you and your accuser. But what if you could see the other as a caring person who is responding anxiously because of a lack of understanding about diabetes? Although you are not being irresponsible, your behavior might be scaring the other person. This mindful change in perspective is a shift from experiencing the situation from inside yourself to seeing it as a curious observer might. From that perspective, your reaction might be to tell the "accuser" that his concern was appreciated but his accusatory tone was not and that he needed to know more about diabetes to understand why you did what you did. This scenario demonstrates another aspect of being mindful: the ability to step out of the drama of the moment and to see the bigger picture. You will learn more about this ability in Chapter 5, in the segment on being emotionally smart.

A mindful person claims maximum control not only in terms of minimizing stress but in maximizing the quality of life. Living mindfully maximizes an individual's opportunity to exercise utmost self-care and to enrich daily life.

It has been said that we are what we think. It has been said, too, that we are what we feel or what we do. Each of these declarations has some merit, but they fail to hit the bullseye. The fact is, that what we think, feel, and do are rooted in what we believe. Think about it. Is there anything you do or don't do that is not linked to what you believe? Consciously or unconsciously, we evaluate each situation in terms of what we believe about the outcome and what we expect to happen.

Decisions are made based on what we believe about our ability to do what is being considered, about how risky or rewarding it might be to do it, and about how much we value doing it. Many young people with diabetes have difficulty maintaining a healthy regimen because they do not believe that taking measures to prevent complications matters at their age. A 19-year-old man is not likely to accept the fact that what he is doing today can have serious consequences many years later.

Thoughts, feelings, and behavior are driven by beliefs. Consequently, being mindful of one's beliefs is vital to self-control and self-care. Most individuals have accumulated beliefs that cause or magnify the stress response and, thus, negatively affect all levels of functioning. Acting on choices that are informed by objective reflection rather than acting habitually on baseless beliefs is taking control of a primary source of stress. In Chapter 8, you will learn the technique of "reframing," the practice of recognizing and replacing faulty beliefs. (The term "frame" has the same meaning as "belief." The term "reframing" refers to changing from one belief to another.) For now, it is important to understand the significance of "believing mindfully," which is being aware, both of the belief that is affecting you and of your ability to change the belief if desired.

What Does Believing Mindfully Mean?

Belief is defined in *The American Heritage Dictionary of the English Language* (3rd edition) as "Mental acceptance of and conviction in the truth, actuality, or validity of something." However, many of the beliefs that we live by are not true, actual, or valid; many have no basis in reality. Despite this truth, most people respond to their beliefs faithfully, even when it hurts.

In *Why We Believe What We Believe: Uncovering Our Biological Need for Meaning, Spirituality, and Truth* (3), neuroscientists Andrew Newberg and Mark R. Waldman describe numerous ways in which the brain biases interpretations of experiences and distorts and constructs its own reality. They suggest that we tend to believe ideas, values, and other information given by family members, by people in positions of power and status, by people in our "in-group," and by individuals who are dramatic and emotional in presenting their point of view. In addition, we are likely to believe information that fits our own expectations, confirms our adopted truths, or benefits our own interests and goals. We are biased, too, to ideas that have an emotional connection. Ideas and values that are supported by a large contingency or that have been published are readily accepted as the truth. The message is clear: we are prone to accept an idea as the truth either because we mindlessly assume that the source is indisputable or because we want to believe it is true. This individualized, biased construction of reality forms many of our beliefs.

Believing mindfully is acting on beliefs that are consciously chosen, beliefs based on informed interpretations of what is happening or derived from fact. It is recognizing that most beliefs, however forceful, are not absolute truths. It is knowing and using the power of choosing a frame that works over a frame that does not work, the power to challenge even the most deeply entrenched biases and distortions of reality.

Why Is Being Mindful Important?

STRESS AND MINDFULNESS

Just as stress is the enemy of diabetes, it can impair the effort to be mindful. Stress is a distraction; it draws attention away from the task at hand. When attention is disrupted by stress, essential information and choices may be missed, and the ability to make sound decisions is hindered. Stress can beat you up in many ways (see Chapters 1 and 2).

The good news is that the connection between stress and mindfulness goes both ways. Being mindful is an antidote to stress. Responding to potentially stressful circumstances in a mindful way reduces, if not eliminates, the chances of a stressful outcome.

DIABETES AND MINDFULNESS

Alice was driving home from work. She was feeling signs of hypoglycemia just before leaving the office, but she thought she would be alright until she got home and could eat something to bring her blood glucose level back to normal. Unfortunately, there was an accident, and she was stuck in traffic for more than an hour. With nothing to elevate her blood glucose level, she became disoriented and unable to function. At some point, another driver realized there was a problem and called for help.

Alice has experienced a very unpleasant and scary event that could have become a chronic worry: "What if it happens again, and no one is there to help me?" Instead, Alice mindfully reviews the range of possibilities that might give her better control. First, Alice decides that she will always check her blood glucose level before driving anywhere, anytime. In addition, she will carry glucose tablets, so that she will always be prepared for similar circumstances. Rather than creating an ongoing stressor, she is confident that driving alone is not a threat if she takes the proper precautions. Being mindful, Alice sees the choices that are possible, and in doing so, she has eliminated a potential source of stress.

Perhaps the worst possible feeling is the feeling of being out of control. Diabetes management is about control, but it is not just about glycemic control. Managing diabetes well is also about controlling your thoughts, feelings, and behavior so that undue stress does not complicate the effort to maintain good blood glucose levels. Being mindful is taking control of one's life in the most useful and meaningful ways. The mindful person is calm but equally wide awake, alert, and ready to handle the routine and difficult aspects of self-care. The mindful individual does not make matters worse by acting on faulty beliefs.

Diagnosed at age 9, Alice had made many mistakes in learning how to take care of herself with diabetes. Unfortunately, her parents would accuse her of being lazy, irresponsible, or even dumb. The belief that these accusations are true was planted firmly in her head. If Alice was not mindful, she would simply have attributed the episode of hypoglycemia to the demeaning notion imposed by her parents. However, thinking mindfully, she realized that the belief was unfounded. Yes, she had slipped up, but not because she was lazy, irresponsible, or even dumb. With this perspective, she learned a lesson and eliminated the possibility of tearing herself down endlessly.

The complications common to diabetes are serious. Preventing their onset should be a high priority. In fact, a reasonable degree of stress about complications is likely to motivate you to do your best to prevent them. However, if the frame for complications is overly pessimistic ("My kidneys and eyes are going to fail, just like they did for my father"), then the fear response will trigger considerable stress and all of its negative consequences.

The fear of complications can trigger other harmful frames such as, "If I *perfectly* manage my diabetes, I can prevent any serious problems resulting from the disease." In Chapter 10, you will learn about the dangers of pursuing perfection. For now, be assured that striving for perfection is a guaranteed stress-producing mental trap. With faulty frames, every facet of diabetes and its care can become a source of mental anguish and a deterrent to effective management.

The individual with diabetes is likely to experience a loss of freedom, particularly with regard to eating. Managing diabetes requires limiting the intake of carbohydrates, which may mean eating favorite foods less often and in smaller amounts. This restriction can be magnified enormously by the frame, "Now that I have diabetes, I will have to give up all of my favorite foods. I can't do this!" With this faulty frame, you will be frustrated and resentful and not in the right state of mind to exercise good care. Frames that are set in absolute terms and include words like "never" or "always" are based on misinformation or a lack of information; they are not true but nonetheless can be very harmful. In fact, individuals with diabetes are not forbidden to have their favorite foods, so long as they are indulging in moderate amounts once in a while.

Behavior change is an essential goal for most individuals who have diabetes. If you are having difficulty managing your diabetes, it is likely that you will need to change your behavior in one or more ways. Behavior change is not just about doing something differently. What you are doing involves how you think and feel; at least, that is how it appears. The fact is that our thoughts and feelings are what we believe about a given situation. (Saying, "I think that . . ." or "I feel that . . ." is saying, "I believe that. . . .")

After being diagnosed with diabetes, Toni is sad and frustrated because she knows it is a serious condition that will require a lot of attention, but she also knows (believes) that it is a manageable disease and that she will take good care of herself.

With the same diagnosis, Fred goes ballistic. He feels threatened by diabetes because he believes that it spells doom. With the combination of anxiety and pessimism, Fred's reaction is contrary to what is needed for making the changes required for good management.

Everyone is familiar with the saying "seeing is believing." By the time you finish reading this book, you should have a mental tattoo that reads, "Warning: believing is seeing." What you believe, you will see, even if it is not there. Beliefs overrule and disprove reality. Think about the placebo effect. There have been numerous studies in which subjects are told that a substance they are given will have a specific effect, and, for many, it has that exact result. But, in fact, they were given a substance that could not cause the effects that were suggested. Having been told to expect a specific outcome and believing in it, the mind and body collaborate to respond accordingly. This way of thinking is important because most of us have a collection of beliefs that are problematic and have no basis in reality—beliefs that can cause serious problems. I call these beliefs "malbeliefs," beliefs that are not only wrong but potentially harmful. A key role of mindfulness is to be alert to the danger of responding to a self-defeating malbelief. Later, you will learn how to identify misbeliefs and malbeliefs and how to overcome them.

As you know, the care of your diabetes is your charge. No one else can do it for you, and being aware of your body is essential to effective self-care. Being mindful eliminates the chance of missing important information conveyed by your body. The mindful person is keenly aware of her or his feelings despite what else is going on.

Acute pain is essential to our survival and well-being. If you accidentally touch a hot pan, the pain is a signal to remove your hand before more damage is done. Similarly, uncomfortable feelings can be a signal that something is wrong and needs to be fixed. If you feel sad, angry, or scared, use the discomfort to trigger a mindful curiosity—beginning with the *mindful questions*:

MQ | *What belief is causing me to feel this way?*

Is the belief valid?

By paying attention, you won't suffer the consequences of reacting to faulty beliefs or overreacting to the feelings that malbeliefs arouse. Being attentive, you are at less risk of being blindsided by some potential danger; there is much less chance of an undesirable surprise. Mindfulness-based stress reduction has been scientifically shown to be effective in reducing stress for a wide variety of medical and psychological conditions, including diabetes.

How Can I Be Mindful?

A tourist in New York City asks someone how she can get to Carnegie Hall. The answer: "Practice, practice, practice." Similarly, the best way to develop the skill of mindfulness is to practice the process over and over again.

GOING TO YOUR CENTER

There are situations in which being *mindful* can be extremely difficult. Perhaps, you are being verbally attacked by someone who is very emotional and somewhat aggressive. Your heart is pounding and your thoughts are racing. If you are going to respond mindfully, you will have to calm yourself down by *centering*. To be centered is to be at the core of your being, the place of calm and strength within you. To attain your center, begin by pausing before you react. Next, take a few deep breaths or more depending on how unsettled you are and how much time you have before you must act. Each time you successfully center yourself, immediately "anchor" the accomplishment with a simple but distinct gesture—such as firmly squeezing your thumb between your index and middle fingers. Over time, the gesture itself can bring you to your center.

Whether you need to center yourself or not, mindfulness is attained with the following steps.

Step 1

The process begins with practicing keen awareness of what you are paying attention to. It begins with periodically asking these *mindful questions*:

MQ	*What am I paying attention to at this moment?*
	Am I missing something that I need to pay attention to?
	Am I in the present?

> *What am I feeling now?*
> *What is it telling me?*

Knowing where you are with regard to each question informs you of any adjustments you need to make to be at your best in any situation. Dealing with a stressful situation requires paying attention to what is happening now. It requires being in the present—not yesterday and not tomorrow. You need to be in touch with your feelings because they can disrupt sound thinking and cause inappropriate behavior. And feelings can give you important information about what is going on.

Step 2

Take the awareness to a deeper level. The next *mindful question* is:

MQ | *Is where I am working*
for me?

One problem is that people get so used to being in a bad place that they do not realize they need to or can change anything. For them, being in a bad place just feels natural. In living mindfully, the task is to break the cycle of automatic thinking and acting by shifting to clear-minded assessment of both the circumstances and the options available.

Step 3

Consider the range of possibilities. If where you are in the moment is working, the obvious choice is to stay with it. However, if where you are is not working, think about the possibilities from which you may choose. The *mindful questions* at this stage are:

MQ | *What can I do to get grounded*
in the present moment?
Is this an opportunity
to reframe a faulty belief?

*What strengths can I draw on
to do my best?*

*What other choices will work better
for me, like getting more information,
delaying a response, or seeking
appropriate help?*

*What can I do to keep this tense
situation from escalating?*

At first, these steps may seem to be too much to learn. You may envision yourself struggling to think of the questions and what to do next. Be assured that with some practice, being mindful will become natural. You have used this process before without thinking of what you were doing. The goal here is to make you aware of the process so that you use it intentionally and with clear purpose. Again, with practice, it will become as natural as many other things that you have been doing effortlessly for a long time.

You are at your regular appointment with your endocrinologist. He has been very stern about your need to lose weight, but you have even gained a few pounds since that last appointment. He is displeased and doesn't hesitate to let you know it. Following the mindful questions in Step 1, you are aware that you feel intimidated and ill at ease. Considering Step 2, it is clear that your distress is not working for you. Guided by your answers to Step 3, take a moment to center yourself and accept responsibility for the weight gain. Then, ask for help. Tell the doctor the circumstances that get you off track, and ask for ideas that will help to achieve your weight goal.

Being Mindful Can Help Manage Diabetes

There are aspects of diabetes self-management for which being mindful can be especially important.

MANAGING HYPOGLYCEMIA
AND HYPERGLYCEMIA MINDFULLY

Your ability to recognize and respond promptly to the signs of hypoglycemia and hyperglycemia is an essential key to managing diabetes and avoiding the discomfort and dangers of extremely low or high blood glucose levels. The symptoms of either condition (see box on page 59) may vary from person to person, and they can be very subtle for someone who has had diabetes for a long time. It is essential to recognize your symptoms and to learn to react promptly. Being *mindful*—in the present and keenly aware of bodily sensations—enables you to maintain control, thereby avoiding a potential crisis.

> *You are busy at work. You feel a bit on edge; you are shaky, but you ignore the discomfort because you are intent on getting some things done. After all, you don't want to annoy the boss, who wants everything done yesterday. However, you remember the commitment to being mindful, and you go through the steps.*

The **mindful questions** are:

MQ | *Is there any reason to be concerned about my blood glucose level at this time?*

Is the uneasiness I am feeling— however slight—a sign of hypoglycemia or hyperglycemia?

If the answer to either question is "yes," check your blood glucose level immediately. Your boss and anyone else would gladly prefer a brief timeout over a call for the paramedics.

Periodically doing a body scan and asking the following **mindful question** can be effective in catching a high or low blood glucose level:

MQ | *In scanning my body, are there any signs that my blood glucose level is too low or too high?*

A body scan simply involves pausing momentarily and going over your body from head to toe to check for signs of a problem. It takes only a few seconds to do; most of the symptoms of highs and lows are physical. Catching a problem before it gains momentum is a real stress-buster. Again, if your answer is "yes" or even "maybe," check your blood glucose level.

EATING MINDFULLY

Eating well most of the time is essential to successful diabetes management. Eating mindfully involves paying attention to what you eat, when you eat, and how you eat. It is being aware of every aspect of eating. Are your mind and body in a good place or are you upset about something? Are there circum-stances that might create a problem, such as a time constraint or the food itself? Are you hungry or have you had enough? Is it time to stop eating? Key *mindful questions* are:

MQ | *Am I free from distraction by other things when I'm eating?*

Am I focused on enjoying all aspects of my meal or snack?

Is my current mood good for making the right choices?

Am I really hungry?

If the answer is "no" to any of these questions, pause, take a deep breath, and do what is necessary to eat mindfully.

There are two common patterns to mindless eating: *1*) eat-ing as a reaction to stress and *2*) eating by habit.

- Perhaps the most frequent response to stress is to eat something that feels comforting or that soothes the feel-ing of uneasiness. In the short run, comfort food works. Eating that bag of chips or that cinnamon bun can be very gratifying in the moment. However, in the big picture, eating sweets or other foods high in calories or carbohydrates—but low in nutritional value—is not only unhealthy, it can heighten your level of stress.

- Eating habitually means eating and drinking the way you always have without considering the pros or cons of the routine—consuming whatever without thinking. Eating too fast or not paying attention to what you are eating can result in eating too much and enjoying it less. Eating mindfully is eating slowly and savoring every bite and every taste. When you eat slowly and pay attention to what you are eating, you are likely to need less food to be satisfied and you will enjoy it to the fullest.

In the last section of this chapter, there are specific directions for practicing being mindful that may make eating a very different and more gratifying experience than you have experienced in the past. The *mindful questions* are:

MQ | *Am I fully enjoying what I am eating? If not, why not? And why am I still eating it?*

Am I in the moment, experiencing this food as much as possible?

MAINTAINING OPTIMISM MINDFULLY

Diabetes can become discouraging. Diabetes is with you 365 days a year; there are no vacations. Diabetes can be especially challenging because of the delicate interactions of glucose, insulin, food, activity, and stress. While it is normal to feel downcast from time to time, it is important to maintain an optimistic attitude (frame) overall, despite the challenges imposed by diabetes. Research has consistently shown that being optimistic is a factor in successfully managing a chronic illness. To this end, the *mindful questions* are:

MQ | *Having diabetes, am I optimistic about the future? If not, what frame is dragging me down?*

Am I locked in, obsessed, with the worst of this disease?

How can I reframe this situation to be enthusiastic and confident about the future despite the diabetes?

How Can I Practice Being Mindful?

The greatest challenge to being mindful is stopping the mindless chatter that takes your attention away from where you want it to be. Acting mindlessly is giving up the power to make alternative choices that are likely to be more beneficial. Choice is power, and power is control, which is the basis of stress management and self-care.

As you practice being mindful, be keenly aware of:
- What you are thinking, feeling, and doing.
- The belief or beliefs that are influencing your thoughts, feelings, and behavior.
- The range of possibilities in every situation.

Here are specific ways to practice being mindful.

1. Put something on your person that will remind you to check where you are in the moment. It is easy to automatically get into a stream of thought and go with it endlessly. You have to train yourself to interrupt the pattern. Carry a lucky charm, put a rubber band on your wrist, or find a relatively flat and smooth stone and carry it in your hand or pocket (as much as possible). This unusual object will get your attention. Use it as a signal to ask the *mindful questions*:

MQ | *What am I paying attention to at this moment?*

> *Is it working for me? If not,*
> *what can I shift my attention to*
> *in order to win here?*

2. If you have a smart phone or digital watch, set it to ring periodically to remind you to practice being mindful. There are apps available for mindfulness training.

3. Take a walk in your neighborhood, a park, or the mall—anywhere will do. Wherever you are, pay attention to what you see, hear, and smell. Pretend you are an artist or photographer, and try to see your surroundings in detail. Create compositions. Note differences in colors, brightness, form, and the spacing of objects. What do you hear or smell? Be curious. Resist the temptation to think about anything that distracts you from being aware of what is happening around you now. Do not judge anything; just be fascinated with everything. Resist the temptation to make judgments; be absorbed, even spellbound, with everything you experience.

4. Practice a meditation from Chapter 15: Mindful Meditation Plus. Keep in mind that although mindful meditation is a valuable component of living mindfully, you practice meditation and you live mindfully.

5. For a snack, eat an apple slowly and mindfully. Take at least 8–10 minutes to finish. Savor every bite. Pay attention only to what is happening in your mouth. Experience the different textures and tastes of the skin, the juice, and the meat of the fruit. Chew the apple slowly; resist the impulse to swallow when what is in your mouth still tastes quite good.

6. Apply this exercise to everything you eat and drink. You will be amazed at the difference when you eat slowly and focus on what you are eating. Be aware of what you are eating, how much you are eating, how your body feels while eating, and even why you are eating. If you eat this

way all the time, you will enjoy your food more and need less to be fully satisfied.

7. Perform a body scan several times a day. Mentally scan your body from head to toe, and note any sensations you are having. Note where the sensation is located. You might coordinate your body scans with checking your blood glucose, which can serve as a reminder to do this task. Doing periodic body scans will help you develop a keen awareness of what is happening in the moment. It also increases your awareness of bodily sensations, a skill that can be very beneficial in managing both diabetes and stress, given that physical discomfort is often the first signal that something is not right.

    As part of this exercise, review the symptoms of hypoglycemia and hyperglycemia often (page 59) to enhance your sensitivity to these conditions.

8. Check your feelings from time to time. Feelings of sadness, fear, or anger can be like a friend, because they tell you there is something that needs your immediate attention. In a state of mindlessness, these same feelings can quickly become your enemies.

Each of these exercises will help you develop the technique of mindfulness, which is essential for living well with diabetes. A goal of the practice is to make mindfulness a natural way of being and not just a technique to use from time to time. A mindful approach to stress control developed at the University of Massachusetts Medical Center is being taught at more than 250 medical centers around the world. Clinical research has shown that mindfulness techniques have a significant impact on mental and physical health, including emotional control. Living mindfully reduces stress and enriches the quality of life. It is a sure path to better glucose management.

SYMPTOMS OF HYPOGLYCEMIA

Lightheadedness
Irritability
Trembling
Confusion
Sweating
Extreme fatigue
Pounding or rapid heartbeat
Slurred speech
Nervousness
Hunger
Poor coordination
Feeling out of your body

SYMPTOMS OF HYPERGLYCEMIA

Dry parched mouth, throat
Sweet or unusual taste
Fatigue, tired all the time
Sleepiness or confusion
Need to urinate
Pain or tingling in extremities
Relaxed feeling

SYMPTOMS OF EITHER CONDITION

Blurred vision
Weakness
Queasiness
Heavy breathing
Frustration
Fatigue
Numbness
Headache
Irritability
Salivation

CHAPTER 4

A Goal-Minded Approach to Behavior Change

Because you are reading this book, it is likely that you want to make some behavior changes. If coping with diabetes has been stressful and your glucose levels have been troublesome, you have made a good decision. This chapter will help you make the changes and make them stick.

The control of stress requires a change in how you think and behave. The change can be immediate ("I will not go to fast food restaurants and eat multilayered cheeseburgers") or may need a series of changes over time ("To lower my A1C, I have to replace some old habits, and it will take some time to get it all together"). But making a change and keeping it going requires more than simply declaring it.

How many times have you decided to change your behavior—with all good intentions—and it never happened or the change did not last very long? Although there are many reasons why good intentions go astray, there is a way to make certain that you get where you want to be. When your goal is to make a change in what you do, there are three steps that are needed to maximize the probability of reaching and maintaining the objective:

1. Set a specific, realistic goal.

2. Make a contract to accomplish the goal.

3. Plan how to achieve the goal.

Why Set Goals?

When you know what you want, you are more likely to get it. That's just common sense, right? The problem is that there is a "knowing" and a "knowing": there is a difference between knowing something in a general way and having specific knowledge about it. You might know that you want to achieve better diabetes management, but to make this goal meaningful requires stating exactly what you mean by better management. Do you mean achieving an A1C of 7% or reducing your A1C by 1% in the next 3 months? A different goal might be to stop drinking soda or to only eat fried foods once every 2 weeks. Setting a workable goal begins with a specific target.

Having chosen a specific objective, success will likely depend on how well you plan to achieve it. Initially, you might not know where to start, or you might understand the problem but not know how to fix it.

An effective strategy for planning how to get from point A to point B is "outcome thinking." Outcome thinking is thinking in reverse order. It is starting with the desired outcome and working backwards to make it happen. If, for example, you have an appointment with your endocrinologist tomorrow, you will probably have a more meaningful experience if you have a goal, an agenda for the encounter, and a plan for achieving a successful outcome. For this situation, the *mindful questions* are:

MQ | *When I am leaving the doctor's office, what would have to have happened to make me feel really good about what took place?*

What is my agenda? What are the issues I want addressed?

Have I covered everything to ensure a successful outcome?

With this mindful approach, you claim a share of the power in the relationship. The agenda is not just the doctor's; it is also yours. Furthermore, you avoid the risk of leaving the doctor's office without getting what you want.

Setting a goal is activating your mental compass. It establishes the direction you want to follow. Focusing on identifying a goal begins with knowing what you want. Once you know your goal or purpose, you have a direction for every action that follows. Clearly, setting a well-defined objective has more meaning and provides more direction for succeeding with your challenge.

How Can I Effectively Set Goals?

IDENTIFY AND PRIORITIZE

The change you want to make may be obvious. If bad eating habits are causing consistently high blood glucose levels, you will want to make changes in the way you eat. If your glycemic management has been problematic, then the immediate goal may not be so clear. Is the answer to exercise regularly or to reduce your carbohydrate intake? If you are not sure why your glucose levels have not been in range, then use the problem-solving model in Chapter 11 to determine what you need to do to achieve better blood glucose levels.

Start by reviewing the list of goals in the table on page 64. As you go through the various goals, place a checkmark beside each one that would benefit you. Then, rank the ones you checked in order of importance to you. Narrow the list to the one goal that is most important. There may be several goals on the list that you want to achieve, but it would be best not to take on too much initially. Even though each goal may be important, you need to be realistic and to rank each one in order of importance. Does one goal have an urgency or importance over another? The objective is to narrow the list to what is most important and most workable. Input from

RANK	GOALS
	Lose weight: lbs by / / (dd/mm/year)
	Exercise (*specify how, when, and for how long*)
	Reduce incidents of hypoglycemia
	Make a significant change in eating habits (*specify the change, e.g., "limiting fried foods to once a month"*)
	Stop smoking by / / (dd/mm/year)
	Broaden my support network
	Eliminate a vulnerability (*identify a specific undesirable situation to get rid of*)
	Practice being mindful (*specify what you intend to do*)
	Practice reframing (*specify what you intend to do*)
	Start meditating (*how, how long, and how often?*)
	Let go of a stressful habit, behavior, grudge, or grievance (*be specific*)
	Enhance my self-esteem (*identify an action that will make you feel better about yourself, e.g., learning something new, such as dancing or playing a musical instrument*)
	Have more fun (*specify what you will do based on what is fun for you, e.g., going bowling once a week or joining a book club*)
	Get more rest (*specify how, e.g., going to bed by 10:00 p.m. at least twice weekly*)
	Any other goal that will reduce your stress and/or improve your diabetes management:

your professional care providers can be particularly helpful in choosing and pursuing a goal.

In setting a goal, start with the *mindful question*:

MQ | *What do I want to change first to reduce stress and manage my diabetes more effectively?*

Once you have identified the goal, the next task is to make the goal as specific as possible.

BE SPECIFIC

It is essential to define each goal as specifically as possible, which usually means identifying your target with numbers. The goal of reducing the frequency of eating fried foods to once a month is more powerful than the goal of eating fried foods less often. With the numbers, you have a way of keeping score, a way of knowing whether you are winning.

Whenever possible, designate a specific period of time for accomplishing a goal. If your objective will take a long time, it probably will be helpful to break it down into smaller segments. So, for example, if your target is to lose 60 pounds in a year, it would be wiser to set a goal of losing 15 pounds every 3 months. This will likely feel more manageable, and you will have the opportunity to celebrate four victories over the year instead of only one.

Use outcome thinking to make the goal even clearer. The *mindful question* is:

MQ | *What will it look like when I accomplish this goal?*

Suppose your goal is to lower your A1C by 2% in 3 months. The answer to the question might be "happier and healthier." If your goal is to lose 30 pounds in 6 months, you might envision a slimmer you. If you have a picture of yourself at or near the desired weight, place it on the refrigerator as an inspiration.

BE REALISTIC

The *mindful questions* are:

MQ | *What is my personal best for this goal?*

Being practical, what might prevent me from meeting my goal?

All things considered, is my goal realistic?

If your A1C has been 10.5% (an average blood glucose of approximately 255 mg/dL), would it be realistic to set your goal as 5.5% (an average blood glucose of approximately 111 mg/dL) in 3 months? This goal might be feasible for some; but for most, this is a setup for disappointment. It might be more realistic to set your goal at 7% (approximately 154 mg/dL). Having achieved your goal, you can make the commitment to get your average glucose levels even lower in the next 3 months. Setting realistic goals requires taking advantage of your strengths and respecting your limitations. It would not be in your best interest to set a goal that puts too much pressure on you. And be sure to engage your healthcare team in the goal-setting process to make certain that your goals are realistic and safe for you.

Achieving a goal can take time and may require a significant behavior change, one that can necessitate some difficult adjustments. Be careful to avoid undue frustration, impatience, and undeserved self-deprecation. Thomas Edison, who is credited with the invention of the light bulb, worked diligently to achieve his goals. One day, a friend stopped at the inventor's workshop. Watching Edison's relentless effort, the visitor could not help but to question why he continued to pursue the objective when he had already failed 1,000 times. Edison replied that he had not failed 1,000 times, but that he was 1,000 steps closer to achieving his goal.

STRETCH

Being realistic does not rule out raising the bar to a reasonable degree. If your goal is to lose 35 pounds, then setting a goal of losing 1–2 pounds a month suggests that you may be kidding yourself about your intention and commitment to the goal. Setting a goal too low will diminish your sense of accomplishment, your enthusiasm, and your self-esteem. You won't feel as good about yourself achieving an easy goal as you would if you stretched some on your target goal and achieved it.

When the desired goal has been defined as specifically and as realistically as possible, the next step in a goal-minded approach to change is to make a contract for reaching the designated target.

Why Make a Contract?

There are several benefits to making a contract to accomplish a goal:

- The process of completing the various parts of a contract often leads to a fuller understanding of all that is involved in pursuing the goal.
- The writing process brings your thoughts to a higher level of consciousness.
- It provides you with a record of the goal and the essential details for accomplishing it, which, in turn, gives you the opportunity to review and reevaluate what you have committed to do.
- Just as athletes sign contracts to perform a certain range of functions for a stated reward, you are signing an agreement to perform a range of activities but for multiple rewards (less stress, better management of your diabetes, better health, and any other rewards you

choose for yourself or that are likely given the goal you have achieved).

Your contract is a vow to yourself to pursue a specific objective in the interest of being better, stronger, and healthier. It serves to solidify the commitment that is essential in making any change in behavior—the more challenging the change, the more important the commitment to yourself.

How Do I Make a Contract?

A model contract is on page 69. A blank contract for your use is on page 70. The steps to making an effective contract are as follows:

1. **State your goal.** Follow the guidelines that are described in detail in the section "How Can I Effectively Set Goals?" (page 63).

2. **Make a plan.** Follow the guidelines described in detail in the section "How Do I Plan to Accomplish a Goal?" (page 71).

3. **Designate a reward for realizing your target objective.** There are guaranteed rewards for accomplishing a goal and for making a healthy behavior change: you will feel better and you will like yourself more. You probably have known the exhilaration of "Yes, I did it!" when a challenge has been met successfully. But for most of us, a more concrete reward provides an additional incentive for staying goal-oriented. Your reward might be buying yourself a new bracelet or some other object of meaning. It might be going to the theater or taking a trip. Giving yourself rewards along the way can be helpful in accomplishing a challenging goal. For example, if you committed to accomplish a goal in 3 months and you are on track for meeting the objective, you might give yourself a modest reward at the midpoint of the contract to reinforce your effort.

4. **Sign and date it.** Make it official and "legal."

MY PERSONAL CONTRACT (*Sample*)

My goal is to:

Lose 15 pounds

By: _3 months from today_

My plan for achieving this goal is to:
(*use as many pages as necessary to complete this vital planning stage*)

- _Eat something sweet only every other day._
- _No fried foods._
- _After checking with my doctor, I will exercise on a treadmill three times a week, starting at 12 minutes and gradually increasing to 30 minutes._
- _Buy good shoes for exercising._
- _Choose to walk rather than ride when possible._
- _Learn as much as I can about the carb content of the foods I eat._
- _Reduce my carb intake by 1/3._

When I accomplish my goal, I will—in addition to the natural rewards of better health, satisfaction, and gratitude—reward myself by:

- _Buy a new dress_
- _Buy a new pair of jeans_

Jane Doe   _4/10/2019_
SIGNATURE   DATE

MY PERSONAL CONTRACT

My goal is to:

_____

_____

_____

_____

By: _____

My plan for achieving this goal is to:
(*use as many pages as necessary to complete this vital planning stage*)

_____

_____

_____

_____

_____

_____

_____

_____

_____

_____

_____

_____

When I accomplish my goal, I will—in addition to the natural rewards
of better health, satisfaction, and gratitude—reward myself by:

_____

_____

_____

_____

_____

_____

_____

SIGNATURE   DATE

When you have completed the contract, sign it and hang it somewhere that will be as visible as possible. The refrigerator, the bathroom mirror, or the inside of your front door are great choices.

How Do I Plan to Accomplish a Goal?

Some goals are relatively simple and easy; others are very complex and more difficult. In either case, there can be pitfalls that make attaining objectives problematic, if not impossible. Generally, good intentions and willpower are not enough to accomplish a goal, especially ones that have repeatedly eluded success. Planning to achieve a goal minimizes the risks of old maladaptive habits and unexpected traps. A well-thought-out plan maximizes the chances of a successful outcome.

The process of planning is basic. Not surprisingly, it begins with two *mindful questions*:

MQ | *Where am I?*
| *Where do I want to be?*

If you wanted to take a car trip to Seattle, Washington, from Baltimore, Maryland, you wouldn't say, "Well, it's northwest of here, so I'll just drive northwest until I get there." Instead, you would look at a map and plan the journey, making decisions about the way to go and where to stop for meals, rest, and sightseeing. The same is true for any goal. Let's say that you weigh 170 pounds and your goal is to lose 15 pounds in 3 months. Let's plan this endeavor.

DRAW A MAP

Throughout this book, you will often be urged to write down your thoughts and ideas. The process of writing takes thinking to another level, and it offers you the opportunity to review and revise what you are thinking. In planning the achievement of a goal, it is even more helpful to draw a map of the journey. Begin the completion of your plan with this *mindful question*:

MQ | *Knowing where I am and where I want to be, what do I have to do to get there?*

Now fill in the map with what you need to do to get there.

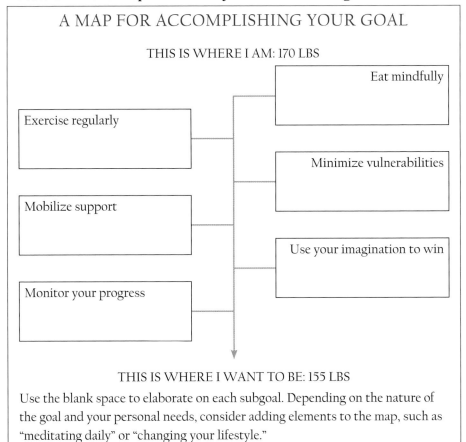

A MAP FOR ACCOMPLISHING YOUR GOAL

THIS IS WHERE I AM: 170 LBS

Eat mindfully

Exercise regularly

Minimize vulnerabilities

Mobilize support

Use your imagination to win

Monitor your progress

THIS IS WHERE I WANT TO BE: 155 LBS

Use the blank space to elaborate on each subgoal. Depending on the nature of the goal and your personal needs, consider adding elements to the map, such as "meditating daily" or "changing your lifestyle."

FILL OUT THE DETAILS

Take the time to plan the journey well. You wouldn't want to be in the middle of nowhere and realize you forgot to bring along an essential item. For the goal of losing weight, I have identified several essential elements to include in the plan, each intended to make the journey a success both in terms of achieving the goal and in making the trip as stress-free as possible. Keep in mind that any of the tools described throughout this book can be included in your plan, depending on your goal and individual needs.

- **Eat mindfully.** First, it is important to know the basics about food, carb counting, and other aspects of what you eat and drink with regard to blood glucose management. Once you know the basics, let's look at eating from a different angle: from how you eat rather than what you eat.

  1. **Learn to eat like a gourmet.** The gourmet—who loves and appreciates quality food—eats mindfully, paying attention to every aspect of the experience. The gourmet always chooses quality over quantity, and favoring large plates with small portions, the gourmet decorates the plate with colorful trimmings to make the presentation as pleasing to the eye as to the palate. Most importantly, the connoisseur eats slowly and savors everything: the tastes, textures, and smells of food and drink and the contrasts and ways that one ingredient brings out the best in another.

     Remember the exercise in Chapter 3 about eating an apple slowly and savoring every bite, giving your total attention to what is happening in your mouth? Hear the sound as you bite into the fruit. Feel the juice flow into your mouth as you penetrate the skin. Be aware of the differences in textures and tastes of the skin and meat of the apple. Carry this experiment over to your next meal. Eat each bite slowly, savoring the various tastes and textures, and do not take the next bite until you have swallowed the last mouthful. Do not wash down what you are chewing when it tastes good. Do not get up to put your dish in the sink while you are chewing the last bite. Be in your mouth; that's where the action is.

When you have learned to eat in this mindful manner, you will enjoy what you eat like never before and you will need less food to be satisfied. Because it may be unnatural for you to do, it may take time to learn. But when you get it, the payoff will be wonderfully gratifying.

The mindful eater avoids two bad habits: eating to remove stress and eating out of boredom. In Chapter 3, you learned about the danger of emotional eating, being compelled to eat and drink to soothe undesirable feelings. It may work for a moment, but in the long run, emotional eating will not only sabotage your diabetes management, it will also cause more stress.

As for eating to avoid being bored, go into mindful mode. A common reason to be bored is to have mindlessly accepted tedium as the only choice. Being bored is not paying attention to the possibilities that are available. If life often feels monotonous, the *mindful questions* are:

MQ | *What can I do to make my free time interesting or exciting?*

Is there something I did in the past that I liked and was good at doing?

Is there a community center nearby that offers an activity of interest?

Doing something creative can be very rewarding, and the challenge of a crossword puzzle or other games can be quite satisfying. Reading and listening to music are other possibilities. Sometimes finding a sense of community through a club or group activity can help. The choices are unlimited. Find what works for you. Do not let life get dull and draw you into bad habits.

If the doldrums persist, consider this possibility:

MQ | *Is it possible I am depressed?*

If the answer is "yes" or "maybe," consult with your doctor about the appropriate treatment.

2. **Be a label hawk.** Although the best choice is to use fresh food products, everyone uses packaged and processed foods to some extent. Pay close attention to the ingredients and nutritional values for commercial foods. Some manufacturers try to trick us into believing their products are healthier than they are. Cookies are one of my favorite treats, so I am always looking for a reasonably healthy cookie. One day, I found an individually wrapped chocolate-chip cookie that looked very appealing and the nutritional values looked just as good . . . or so I thought. As I began to open the wrapping at home, I realized that the serving size for the stated nutritional values was for one-third of the cookie, which meant that the total values were three times what was on the label. Another cookie I had latched onto listed soy butter as an ingredient. I learned later that it was the manufacturer's term for partially hydrogenated soybean oil, an absolute no-no.

If the ingredients and the nutritional values on a package do not jell, put the package back on the shelf. If the product is still tempting, consider, as I did, contacting the manufacturer's customer service to verify the nutritional information. If you are going to eat at a chain restaurant, check its website for postings of the nutritional values of their offerings. One chain's "low-fat chicken noodle soup" contains 1,400 mg sodium, 58% of the recommended daily intake. The information may not be available, but give it a try.

- **Exercise.** The physical benefits of exercise are numerous. Strengthening the heart, toning the muscles and bones, burning calories, and lowering blood pressure are important rewards for exercise. Even moderate exercise reduces blood glucose levels. Furthermore, research suggests that exercise reduces the risk of some cancers. Studies have shown, too, that regular physical exercise can reduce the risk of developing Alzheimer's disease by up to 50%. What's more, exercise can also slow further deterioration in individuals who have already started to develop cognitive problems.

  Although the physical benefits of exercise are more commonly known, the mental and emotional benefits of regular exercise are considerable. Being physically active reduces stress by distracting from worry and releasing physical tension. Studies indicate that individuals who exercise regularly feel better, have more energy, are in a better mood, feel more relaxed, and sleep better. Furthermore, people who exercise regularly tend to be less susceptible to depression.

  Keep in mind that you do not have to exercise vigorously. Studies of cultures whose citizens tend to live the longest have found that high-energy exercise is not a factor. Their primary source of exercise is walking. Know that whatever you are capable of doing—however moderate—will be beneficial. Of course, if you have a physical or medical condition, check with your physician before starting an exercise program.

- **Minimize vulnerabilities.** Identify conditions or situations that may weaken or thwart your plan. Then, use any of the perspectives and skills presented throughout this book to neutralize them. The *mindful questions* are:

MQ | *What circumstances can be a barrier to achieving my goal?*

What do I need to do to eliminate this barrier?

For example, if you are pessimistic about your ability to control your food intake to lose weight, you need to reframe (Chapter 8) that negative belief or beliefs. Some individuals who are dieting become discouraged at the prospect of reducing their food intake for weeks or months. Their frame might be, "I can't do it. Every time I try, I get frustrated and give it up." A positive reframe to consider is, "One day at a time." The message is simple and straightforward: "I don't have to do it for 6 weeks or 2 months; I just have to do it today."

If your work makes it difficult to eat regularly or it often puts you in fast food restaurants, use the problem-solving model in Chapter 11 to find a way around what is in your way.

Some lifestyles make losing weight difficult (Chapter 7). Lifestyles that include eating fatty foods, drinking too much alcohol, or eating fast food too often will sabotage your efforts. If your lifestyle works against your goal, then your plan must include whatever changes are needed to reduce or eliminate each barrier. If, for example, you drink a couple of six packs of beer each week and giving that up will be very difficult, consider an incremental reduction. Make the commitment to reduce your intake by half the first month and by half again the second month. Moderate adjustments over time are likely to be more acceptable.

Excessive stress is a vulnerability for many individuals who are trying to lose weight. Stress and overeating go with one another. Identify each source of stress, and use the skills throughout this book to eliminate or reduce them as much as possible. Reframing, meditation, and humor are just a few of the possibilities for getting a stressor off your back.

Be mindful of any external barriers to achieving your goal. The *mindful questions* are:

MQ | *Are there any external barriers to achieving my goal?*

What can I do to eliminate these barriers?

For example, if your goal is to lose weight, some medications may work against you. Some people find that taking insulin can make losing weight difficult. One problem that resulted from the advent of the insulin pump was the ease of using boluses to compensate for excessive eating. This approach may work in the short run; but over time, this method will lead to weight gain.

Beware of a goal that depends on someone else to achieve it. Because you cannot control the behavior of others, it can be risky depending on someone else to accomplish an objective. If your goal is to walk one mile every morning but you only do it if your neighbor walks with you, then you have forfeited control of the outcome.

Holidays can be a barrier to losing weight. Thanksgiving, Christmas, the New Year, and other special times can make it difficult to eat sensibly. Having a big, rich meal occasionally is not likely to be harmful because you can compensate in various ways, including eating more conservatively before and after, exercising more than usual during the holiday season, and, perhaps, making an adjustment in the medication you are taking. The problem during the holidays is that the celebration becomes an ongoing feast over many days, which in addition to punishing the body may lead to giving up on your desire to achieve your weight-loss goal.

The purpose for being mindful of vulnerabilities is to anticipate and eliminate any barriers to accomplishing your goal (see Chapter 12). This approach uses the old saying, "Know thine enemy." When you know there is an obstacle ahead, you have the choice of taking another route to get where you want to be.

- **Mobilize a support network.** Managing diabetes can be demanding; having healthy, caring support can be comforting and even essential. There can never be too much support (so long as it is truly supportive as opposed to someone beating on you because they are uninformed about managing diabetes).

Research on the outcome of medical cases, such as recovery from a heart attack, has consistently shown that patients who had the support of significant others tended to have better outcomes than individuals who lacked the help and encouragement of others. It makes perfect sense given the natural need to be connected with others, to feel worthy of the care of others, and to be reassured that significant others can be trusted to respond if necessary.

Support is what you get from someone other than yourself. Being independent is good up to a point, but there are times when each of us will have to depend on someone else to get through a difficult situation.

For example, having good support can be extremely important when a blood glucose level is so low that self-care becomes difficult or impossible. The more people in your life who know the symptoms of hypoglycemia, the better. Interdependence is a strength not a weakness.

One way to mobilize a support network is to educate the people on whom you can rely. A frequent complaint I hear from people who have diabetes is dealing with people who mean well but continually dump their misinformation about diabetes on others. In at least one culture, diabetes is commonly referred to as the "sugar disease," implying that sugar is the cause of the ailment and all of its struggles. Inform people in your support network about hypoglycemia, hyperglycemia, carbs, and glucose and dispel myths, such as having diabetes means you cannot eat anything that contains sugar. Do whatever you can to dispel their fears about it. Irrational reactions to the behavior of someone with diabetes are often the result of undue fear and misguided concerns.

Another way to organize support is to participate in a diabetes support group. Your local hospital or diabetes clinic may sponsor a group. If not, consider starting a group by suggesting the idea at your medical center or to an endocrinologist. A support group not only provides you with the opportunity to learn from others who have diabetes, it also gives you the opportunity to be of assistance to them. In writing about the value of a caring support team, I am reminded of working with several patients who were facing serious and scary medical procedures. A number of strategies can help patients feel more secure. In addition to interventions with the hospital medical staff, I have encouraged patients to organize a "goon squad." The squad consisted of significant others who agreed to be available at any time of day or night to talk by telephone for as long as the patient wanted. I was a member of each goon squad, the name coming from the belief that one would have to be a goon to agree to be awakened in the middle of the night to talk. Friends of the patient were eager to join up, which was comforting to the patient on many levels.

- **Imagine winning.** Many athletes and performers use their imagination to enhance their routines. Research has shown that what we tell ourselves and envision has an impression on the mind and body. If your goal is to lose 15 pounds and you have a picture of yourself at about that weight, post it where you will see it as often as possible. If you don't have a picture at your goal weight, create an imaginary one in your mind's eye. In either case, see the image of yourself at your goal weight often.

- **Monitor progress regularly.** If you were on a long road trip, you would automatically check your progress from time to time, wouldn't you? Are you on the right route? With so many miles to go, should you call ahead and say that you will be late? Knowing where you are in relation to where you are going is empowering; it gives you more control of the situation.

There are a number of possibilities for monitoring the goal of losing 15 pounds in 3 months. Take a few minutes at the end of each day or week to ask yourself these *mindful questions*:

MQ | *How did I do today? This week?*

Did I fall off my plan anywhere along the way?

> ### *What can I do to prevent that from happening again?*

Another possibility is to set interim goals. How about checking at the end of each month to see if you have lost about 5 pounds, which would mean that you are in line with losing 15 pounds in 3 months? In addition, periodically weighing yourself would be helpful. However, it raises the question of how often to weigh yourself. For some, weighing in every day at the same time can be beneficial because it provides an opportunity to make adjustments for that day or the next. For others who tend to worry or dwell on things too much, it can be more helpful to weigh in less often. Remember, one of the principles of goal setting is to be realistic, which means, in part, knowing and respecting who you are. The *mindful question* is:

MQ | *Is what I expect of myself consistent with who I am?*

Obviously, when the answer is "no," the plan has to be reconsidered and adjusted. Some people do better with high expectations and others with less. It's not a matter of right or wrong; it is an issue of individual differences.

Whatever your goal might be, it is important to periodically check how you are doing. Tracking progress is keeping score. Periodically checking where you are in relation to the goal gives you the opportunity to make adjustments, if necessary.

Imagine you are a pilot landing an airplane. You see the runway (your goal), and if you are too far to the left or right, you make the necessary adjustments. To see if your approach is too slow or too fast, you check your instruments (weight scale and glucometer). Just as the pilot lands his craft mindfully, a goal-minded approach to behavior change will land you safely on your designated runway.

What If the Plan Is Not Working?

MAKE NECESSARY ADJUSTMENTS

Remember, choice is power. To claim the power of choice requires a high level of flexibility. Being flexible means being able to change your mind in response to what is happening and remain open to considering other options when your plan is not working. Consider yourself like the bamboo that bends with the wind without breaking.

When the plan is not working, your task is to identify the glitch or glitches and fix or find a way around them. The *mindful questions* are:

MQ

> *What is getting in my way?*
>
> *What do I need to change to accomplish the goal?*
>
> *What part of my plan is not working? What choices do I have to overcome it?*
>
> *What strengths or resources can I draw on to make this work?*
>
> *Do I need to rethink the goal?*

Suppose, for example, that you had planned to go to a health club every other day to work out on a treadmill, but you are finding it too difficult to follow the schedule. Consider an alternative routine for the days you cannot get to the health club, perhaps a brisk 20- to 30-minute walk before breakfast or supper. There are numerous, reliable sources for advice about exercising and diabetes. Check the list of websites and apps on pages 327–328. If, for example, you try diabetes.org (American Diabetes Association), look for the "search" symbol (Q) in the upper right corner of the homepage and type in "exercise."

REASSESS YOUR MOTIVATION

If your plan is not working and you cannot identify what is wrong, check your motivation for pursuing the goal. Is the goal someone else's agenda? Are you trying to please someone else, and, in reality, it is a low priority for you? Here are some *mindful questions* that will help you determine whether lack of motivation is the problem:

MQ | *Do I believe I can achieve the goal?*

Do I value achieving the goal?

Is the reward for succeeding greater than the risk of trying?

If the answer to any of these questions is "no," then motivation is likely the problem. Of course, the next step is to understand why your answer to one or more of the *mindful questions* is negative. Why do you doubt that you can attain the goal? Why don't you value reaching the goal? How concerned are you about the risk regarding your stated objective?

A reason for setting and contracting to achieve a goal is to solidify your commitment to the change you have chosen, and degree of commitment is directly related to the degree of motivation. If you are not motivated to make the change, you won't be committed to make it happen—and it won't happen.

STUCK? GET HELP

If you are stuck, get help. Your healthcare team is there to help you set safe and realistic goals and overcome challenges to meeting your objectives. There is no shame in asking for help; the shame is in needing help and not asking for it. You will know when you are stuck. If losing 15 pounds in three months is the goal and it doesn't happen, then you are stuck. You may have a sense of what the problem is and seek help accordingly. You may sense that the diet you have formulated is not working, in which case consider consulting a dietitian. If you are taking medication that tends to work against losing weight, you might consult with your physician about a possible change in your medication regimen. If you are struggling with anxiety or depression, a consultation with someone in the mental health field will likely be beneficial. If you do not have a sense of what the problem is, then you might want to consult a diabetes specialist. Sometimes, all you need may be the backing of your support team.

Why Is Commitment Important?

Making a commitment is making a vow or a pledge to do something. However, without genuine intention, the act is useless. When the commitment is deeply valued, it becomes the sense of conscientiousness that makes the difference when the mission is at its most difficult. It becomes a driving force when you are at a crossroads between giving up and pushing on despite the discomfort of doing so.

The multibillion-dollar self-help publishing industry rides on the difficulty so many people have with keeping a commitment. Most self-help books have some ideas that are beneficial to adopt and practice—suggestions that could lead to positive gains for most readers. Buyers, often captured by the promises of the title and back cover, are excited by the expectation of overcoming whatever troubles them. The problem is that they may not be willing or ready to do the grunt work that is required. It has been said, "Everyone wants to go to heaven; nobody wants to die." Everyone wants to grow, to overcome hardships, and to change anything that causes stress and pain, but fewer are willing to maintain the discipline and to endure the discomfort of changing old patterns and experiences.

Yes, it can be difficult and emotionally painful to change behaviors, even when the habit you want to change has been very unkind to you. We become attached to things: to people, to objects, and to beliefs. And when we get attached to something, we tend to hold on tenaciously, no matter what.

CHAPTER 5

Being Emotionally Smart

E motion can be defined as a conscious state of feeling in reaction to what one believes is happening and what it means to the affected person. Visiting the zoo, you might have a feeling of joy at seeing your favorite animals at play. However, if you are visiting the zoo and see a loose tiger, then you will perceive danger and feel fearful. In this case, the feeling is adaptive because it arouses the fight-or-flight response, which maximizes the chance of surviving an encounter with the beast. The response enables you to make vital adjustments in reaction to the crisis you are facing. However, if a mouse ran across your path and you felt the same fear, then the fight-or-flight response is maladaptive. In this example, the feeling of fear has mind and body responding inappropriately to a harmless creature.

Emotions can have a powerful impact on one's behavior. Many individuals who have a fear of mice have told me they would have to leave the room if they were told that a mouse had been seen there recently.

Alice is 42 years old and has had type 2 diabetes for 3 years. Her glucose levels have been erratic, and her endocrinologist has recommended that she switch from oral medications to insulin. The doctor's advice provoked Alice's belief that it was a sign of impending doom, and the fear led her to strongly resist making the change. The fear led to behavior that was not in her best interest.

Adam has a similar profile. His doctor also recommended that he shift to insulin to improve his diabetes management. Adam responded to the suggestion as a positive change; he did not believe it was a threat. He felt optimistic, and he quickly agreed to start using insulin.

Two people in similar situations have different beliefs and very different reactions: Adam's was positive, and Alice's was negative. When the intensity and extent of an emotion are not consistent with what is happening, the reaction will be unfavorable. In the face of real danger, fear is adaptive; the feeling is an appropriate defense against perceived danger, activating the fight-or-flight response. The fear that many with type 2 diabetes experience with regard to switching from oral medications to insulin is maladaptive because it is usually based on the belief that the change in treatment is a negative sign: bad news. Consequently, many individuals who would benefit from making the change avoid it and deny themselves the best care possible.

Chapter 3 presents two distinct concepts: 1) that you live by what you believe and 2) that what you believe in any given situation determines how you will think, feel, and act under the circumstances. You learned that when you can recognize that a belief is not working for you, then you can change the belief to one that does work. With this action, you are taking mindful control of how you think, feel, and act. You are using the power of mindfulness to control your feelings and keep stress at a minimum.

In the discussion of being emotionally smart, you will learn that an emotion can incite an undesirable reaction unless you exercise the power of choosing how you are going to act regardless of the feeling or emotion. You will learn that you can choose how you will react to a feeling. Being aware of the emotion and mindfully choosing how to react gives you control of what happens next.

Some individuals are ruled by their feelings. They tend to act on their emotions without thinking about the consequences. Negative feelings—powerlessness, frustration, anger, anxiety, sadness, or fear—dominate their thoughts and actions. The resulting behavior is mindless, and the consequences are stressful, sometimes dreadfully so. Managing your feelings is essential for keeping stress at a minimum, managing your diabetes, and determining the quality of your life.

What Does Being Emotionally Smart Mean?

Being emotionally smart is part of living mindfully. It is about recognizing and accepting your feelings and having the ability to manage them constructively. Faced with intense feelings of anxiety, desire, sadness, or anger, the emotionally smart person transcends the feeling and mindfully chooses the best possible response under the circumstances. The one who is emotionally unaware reacts blindly and, often, at great risk. Not being emotionally smart can have many unfavorable consequences for diabetes management.

Being emotionally smart does not mean controlling how you feel. It does not mean never feeling angry, anxious, or sad. It means not giving in to the feeling; it means finding a way to rise above the discomforting emotion. Being emotionally smart is recognizing when a feeling is pushing or pulling you to act inappropriately. It is about making an informed choice that overrides the urge to act wrongly. Being emotionally smart is more about controlling your reaction to an emotion than it is about controlling the emotion. When a reaction to an emotion is positive, it is adaptive; when a feeling provokes a negative reaction, it is likely to have unfavorable consequences.

How Can I Prevent Maladaptive Reactions to My Emotions?

Many of the emotional experiences that have been given their own names are variations on a short list of primary feelings. Although there may not be a universal agreement on which emotions are primary, it is reasonable to identify powerlessness, anxiety, fear, anger, sadness, desire, and humiliation as the core feelings with a high risk for causing maladaptive behavior. With these feelings, an unfavorable reaction is probable if responded to mindlessly. Remember that having the feeling may be appropriate, but the reaction to it can be wrong. You may have reason to be angry at someone, but that does not give you the right to do harm to another.

Emotions have a powerful influence on how things are experienced. They tend to incite action, often overwhelming reason. The action that is provoked has been programmed, in part, by the evolutionary history of humanity, particularly the basic survival mechanisms of the fight-or-flight response. Feelings have been programmed, too, by each individual's personal experiences. A child who was traumatized in the process of getting immunization shots may have an intense fear of injecting insulin many years later. Being emotionally smart is recognizing that the reaction to a feeling is being driven by a program that is not relevant to the current situation and then to make a mindful decision about what to do next.

It is important to understand that reactions to emotions can be adaptive or maladaptive. The same feeling can have a positive or a negative effect, depending on the situation. When the reaction to a feeling is adaptive, the outcome is beneficial. If you are annoyed at someone for being inconsiderate of your needs and you firmly inform him that his behavior is not acceptable, then the anger has enabled you to assert yourself and set a boundary with the other. When feelings trigger maladaptive reactions, the results are stressful or worse. If someone you cared about was inconsiderate of your needs and your annoyance turned to fury, compelling you to end the relationship, then the reaction was maladaptive; it was a lose-lose outcome. Because maladaptive reactions to feelings can be so stressful and otherwise undesirable, the main focus in this chapter is on the emotions that tend to produce unfavorable results.

What makes a specific feeling either adaptive or maladaptive? A reaction to a feeling is adaptive when it is appropriate to the circumstances that provoked the emotion. An adaptive reaction is mindful, and it is consistent with reality; the manner in which the feeling is expressed is in proportion to what provoked it.

Feelings such as joy, pride, acceptance, and love generally result in adaptive reactions. However, even these emotions can cause an unfavorable outcome. Many things that are pleasurable should not be done under certain circumstances. Activities that produce positive feelings are positive so long as they are not done to excess. Having a piece of candy may be joyful, but having a box of candy becomes a problem.

A strong feeling of trust can inspire love and devotion, but blind trust can have devastating consequences. Love can be more lust than adoration. It is appropriate to mourn a loss— the loss of a loved one, a function, a job, or any personal loss. However, it is maladaptive to exaggerate each and every loss and then to grieve excessively.

In Chapter 3, you learned to use your feelings as a signal to pause and reflect on the belief that has stirred the emotion. With this technique, you avoid the risk of acting on the basis of a faulty belief. In being emotionally smart, your emotions also serve as a signal to pause to reflect on how to react to the feeling. During the pause, reflect on these *mindful questions*:

MQ | *Is the belief that is causing me to feel this way consistent with reality? Is it true?*

Is the intensity and extent of what I am feeling consistent with what is happening?

Have I put the feeling to the test of reason?

Do I understand what happened or do I need to get more information?

Although I feel like I want to strike back or give up, what can I do to make the best of this situation?

What can I do to bring about a win-win outcome?

As you reflect on these questions, here are some important aspects of the emotional experience to keep in mind:

- Having a feeling is never wrong. The brain is wired to react automatically to a variety of stimuli. How you feel is not in your control, but how you respond to a feeling can be managed mindfully.
- Acting mindlessly on a feeling can be very wrong and often dangerous. An automatic, impulsive response to an emotion puts you at risk of reacting for the wrong reason or overreacting to what has taken place. (Road rage is an example of the danger of impulsively acting on a feeling.)
- In the way that a color has many shades, emotions have a range of intensity. Anger, for example, is a continuum of experiences ranging from being mildly annoyed to being enraged. In most situations, it is alright to express annoyance or frustration, but it is rarely reasonable to act on the feeling of rage (see the box on page 95).
- The connection between emotions and stress goes both ways, not in just one direction. Emotions can be stressful, and stress can arouse emotions. The discomfort of stress can provoke a range of feelings, including anger, anxiety, sadness, and desperation, and these feelings, in turn, are stressful.

How Will Being Emotionally Smart Help Manage My Diabetes?

Diabetes care requires continual vigilance, monitoring, decision making, and problem solving. All of these tasks are done under the threat of an unexpected (and often undeserved) change in blood glucose levels and the threat of various serious complications. It is understandable that dealing with diabetes can generate a range of intense feelings. There are times when you may feel that managing your diabetes is just too overwhelming.

Few experiences can be more stressful than losing control of one's feelings. We see the extreme examples in the newspaper and on the evening news when people get enraged and hurt someone. But very few of us escape the regretful experience of acting impulsively and either hurting someone's feelings or "shooting oneself in the foot." Being the perpetrator or the target of uncontrolled, negative feelings is stressful, and stress is an enemy of diabetes management. Stress has unhealthy effects on the body and the mind, effects that directly or indirectly impair glucose management. If the connection between stress control and diabetes management is not clear to you, review Chapters 1 and 2. In addition to causing the stress response, emotional stressors can have other unfavorable effects on diabetes management.

Diabetes requires a great deal of attention and decision making, and nothing can muddle the ability to perform these functions more than irrational anxiety or fear. Like the anxiety of seeing a tiger loose at the zoo, anxiety about having diabetes motivates you to take good care of it, even though it may be unpleasant to do so. However, excessive anxiety is disruptive, causing a state of mind opposite of the calmness that is necessary for clear, objective decision making.

Diabetes comes with its own set of worries and fears. Many people worry about reactions to low blood glucose, long-term complications, and the impact that self-management will have on their lives. When the reactions to these worries are excessive, they become serious deterrents to good self-care. For example, some people who are fearful of hypoglycemia try to keep their blood glucose levels higher all the time by cutting back on medications and exercise and by eating more. Some may binge when they sense the slightest sign of low blood glucose. If you think of coping with diabetes in terms of the fight-or-flight response, such a reaction makes sense. To many people with diabetes, a low blood glucose level is a perceived danger. Thus, if you fear hypoglycemia, you may avoid or "flee" this threat by going in the opposite direction and keeping your blood glucose levels high. Unfortunately, this reaction is not necessarily healthy for you in terms of potential long-term complications. Similarly, the fear of insulin injections might lead to the rejection of an essential treatment.

Anxiety is not all bad; it has a useful purpose. Worrying can help lead you to find a solution to a problem. If you are worried about what you are going to eat at the annual office picnic and your concern leads to a positive solution, then the anxiety was actually helpful. However, if you are constantly worried and anxious, then there is a problem that needs to be resolved. You will learn some possible causes for feeling anxious as you continue with this chapter.

Take notice if your worrying evolves into fear, compelling you to avoid situations and people who are integral to your health and well-being. People whose worry about hypoglycemia has turned into a full-blown fear may begin to avoid activities like driving or avoid doing anything that takes them too far away from home. Fear can be a serious problem for people with diabetes because it can be disruptive to effective self-care.

Anger can distract you from doing what needs to be done. Being occupied with feelings of annoyance, resentment, or fury prevents thoughtful consideration of what needs attention. Anger can lead to inappropriate behavior that makes the situation even more troublesome. Have you ever eaten something

A GUIDE TO MALADAPTIVE EMOTIONS

ANGER* is a feeling of displeasure that can be viewed on a continuum from being annoyed, frustrated, furious, or enraged to feeling hostile. The more intense the anger, the greater the risk of inappropriate behavior.

ANXIETY* is a sense of apprehension and worry, often in response to an imprecise, unknown threat. Many mental disorders are rooted in anxiety, including obsessive-compulsive behavior and posttraumatic stress disorder.

DESIRE* ranges from wanting or wishing for something, to the more troublesome longing or craving for what promises to be enjoyable or pleasurable, to various devastating addictive behaviors.

FEAR is an intense emotional response to the perception of danger. A PHOBIA* is an irrational and excessive fear of a threat, real or imagined. PANIC* is a sudden, overpowering feeling of terror, usually involving palpitations, and its cause may not be apparent.

SADNESS is a sense of sorrow or unhappiness that varies in intensity, including MELANCHOLY* (lingering or habitual sadness) and DEPRESSION* (gloom, with a sense of inadequacy, hopelessness, and helplessness).

SHAME (often confused with GUILT, which is a remorseful awareness of having done something wrong) is a strong sense of unworthiness, of being a deplorable person. With shame, self-blame is the default frame when anything goes wrong.

These feelings, when prolonged and persistently troubling, are the basis for various mental disorders.

---

you didn't want to eat just to spite someone who has angered you? Anger can be very stressful.

Many people are angry about their diabetes. You might be mad at having to constantly monitor your eating habits. You may get frustrated with not getting positive results when you have been trying so hard to manage your diabetes. You may simply be angry at having diabetes—experiencing that nagging feeling of "why me?" If you again think back to the fight-or-flight response, you can gain some perspective into your anger. Remember that diabetes is a potential threat to your health and general well-being. So your anger can motivate you to fight the danger with all your might.

A feeling of sadness can disrupt self-care in several ways. Energy level generally coincides with one's mood. Feeling low is usually a mental and physical experience. Lacking both the right mood and energy to do something that is less than pleasant, such as checking your blood glucose level, is not likely to motivate doing what is necessary. The deeper the sadness, the more the emotion interferes with effective diabetes management. At the extreme end of the spectrum of sadness, the state of depression, individuals can be completely unable to take care of themselves.

Feeling down and discouraged is not conducive to doing what is needed for effective diabetes management. A sad mood may lead to neglecting responsibilities, particularly when what has to be done is not pleasant. Diabetes care will suffer in the short term, but prolonged despondence may lead to a state of melancholy or depression, making effective self-care very difficult. (It is estimated that a person with diabetes is four to five times more likely to become depressed than someone who does not have the disease.)

Desire, the urge to do or have something, is a common experience. A wholesome desire motivates the pursuit of worthy goals and successes. For some, however, the desire for something that is unhealthy or immoral can be irresistible. Resisting the yearning for the fried chicken or pie à la mode or some other treat—especially when others are having some—is a frequent struggle for people with diabetes.

Developing the ability to resist temptations, to oppose the desire to do something that is likely to have a bad outcome, will help you maintain good glucose levels. How often are you tempted to eat something that will make your blood glucose level soar? How many times have you had an irresistible urge to eat too much? Are you too busy to take good care of yourself because you have some material ambition? Everyone struggles at times with self-indulgence or the need for gratification, even when we know there will be consequences. Controlling the urge for immediate gratification is an important component of being emotionally smart; it is vital to successfully managing diabetes. As you practice being emotionally smart, you will be able to have the long-term satisfaction of taking the best care of yourself by resisting the temptation of short-term gratification. You will experience the joy of exercising self-control—of having avoided suffering the consequences of giving in to an unhealthy urge.

Blame is a curse on the blamer and the blamed. Individuals with diabetes often experience feelings of guilt or shame that are associated with self-condemning beliefs—an episode of severe hypoglycemia may lead to thinking you are a failure and cannot do anything right. Blaming yourself for mistakes or misfortune has a downward spiraling effect, stirring corresponding feelings of despair and defeatism. Blaming others for your misfortune has the same negative impact, arousing feelings of resentment and victimization. These emotions are not conducive to successful diabetes care. To avoid blaming oneself or another does not mean to deny responsibility or accountability for a wrongdoing. Blame implies condemnation, a sharp reprimand for an action. Unfortunately, the rebuke is often directed to the person rather than his or her behavior. A healthy way to address a wrongdoing is to acknowledge it happened, to appropriately designate responsibility, and to *mindfully* do what is necessary to prevent a recurrence.

Being emotionally smart involves having empathy for the feelings of others. There is no doubt you have been the target of someone's discontent, the object of another's anger or hostility. You may recall how such an incident stirred feelings of hurt and resentment. While the feeling is understandable, acting on it mindlessly will most likely have ill effects.

At work, Brian had injected his usual dose of insulin in anticipation of eating lunch. Shortly afterward, there was a fire drill. Brian was one of the company's fire wardens, and he had responsibilities that distracted him from eating as he had intended. Brian's blood glucose level dropped so low that he became disoriented. The paramedics were summoned, which was another disruption to production. Later, despite the fact that he had put duty over his self-interest, he was reprimanded and warned that another disruption to operations would result in action against him. Frustrated, he was torn between quitting or forcefully protesting his unfair treatment. Reacting to his anger by quitting or arguing with his supervisor would have been counterproductive.

Being emotionally smart, Brian knew that sometimes the best way to control one's own feelings is to have empathy for the feelings of the other. He realized that the company's managers had been under a lot of pressure to increase production. Although he thought the reprimand was unfair, he understood that his manager was acting out of fear, which caused him to overreact. Brian decided he would use his conflict-resolution skills in a meeting with his manager later on (see Chapter 6).

How Do I Become Emotionally Smart?

Three essential aspects of being emotionally smart are 1) *mindfully* controlling an intense feeling that otherwise might lead to a regretful incident, 2) having the ability to resist temptations and cravings, and 3) having a mindful regard for the feelings of others. A review of these approaches to being emotionally smart follows.

TRANSCENDING MALADAPTIVE EMOTIONS

There are five steps to transcending—rising above—an intense emotion.

Step 1. Awareness—Being aware of a feeling is essential to having control of what happens next. The sooner a feeling is recognized, the better. Practicing being mindful will increase your ability to recognize what you are feeling more quickly. Even if you cannot identify the emotion specifically, any sense of emotional discomfort is a signal to follow this process.

Step 2. Pausing—Reactions to feelings tend to be automatic and fast, especially when the feeling is associated with the perception of danger. Any perceived threat—real or imagined—will set off the fight-or-flight response. Avoid acting impulsively. Pausing allows you the opportunity to mindfully consider the best options for a favorable outcome. Being frustrated by the hostess who keeps insisting that you eat that piece of pie you don't want may make you feel like pushing the pie into her face, but this is not really an option. Pausing will help you get past the moment of distress and allow time to think about what to do. Unless you are in a situation that is a real threat to your well-being, pausing upon recognizing a negative feeling is essential. Certainly, if the threat is real, then it is vital to act instinctively to survive the danger.

Step 3. Acceptance—Do not feel guilty for having an emotion. Generally, we do not have control of what we feel. The emotions originate in the limbic system, a primitive part of the brain primarily concerned with survival. Reason, planning, learning, and memory are functions of the neocortex, the most recently evolved part of the human brain. When circumstances trigger an emotional reaction, the limbic system is activated before the neocortex (the reasoning part of the brain), so it is not your fault that you feel scared, angry, or sad at times. It is not in your control. What happens next is your choice.

Individuals whose undesirable emotions are rooted in psychological issues tend to act on the feelings inappropriately. Some are characteristically prone to a particular emotion. For example, some individuals are angry or sad a lot of the time. When there is a pattern of emotion-driven negative behavior, professional assistance may be necessary to overcome the problem.

Step 4. Reflection—Acting mindfully is always a factor in achieving self-control, stress control, and managing diabetes. If you are reacting to a feeling, the *mindful questions* at this point are:

> *I feel ——————, and I am tempted to ——————, but what would happen if I act on my feeling?*
>
> *What choices do I have that will work the best for me?*
>
> *For each choice, what are the probable consequences and at what cost?*
>
> *What is the smart thing to do now? Would I benefit by reframing this situation?* (See Reframing, Chapter 8.)

At some time after having resisted the impulse to act inappropriately, there is an opportunity to explore what caused you to have the feeling. Consider these *mindful questions*:

MQ

> *What was the stimulus/trigger that caused me to feel so ——————?*
>
> *What frame or frames caused the troublesome feeling?*
>
> *How can I reframe the experience if it happens again?*

The answers to these questions can lead to understanding and preventing a similar problem in the future.

The object is to choose the response that is likely to produce the best consequences at the lowest cost. For example, the person who felt like smashing the pie into the face of the hostess has several choices with differing outcomes: *1)* he could be physically aggressive and smash the pie into her face, *2)* he could be verbally aggressive and curse at the hostess for her insensitivity, or *3)* he could firmly inform the hostess that although she means well, she needs to respect his refusal of the pie. Obviously, the latter choice has the best chance of producing a positive outcome. The consequences and costs of the aggressive options are apparent. Chapter 6: Essential People Skills presents a range of techniques for resolving disagreements and other intense conflicts.

Step 5. Choose and Act—The best choice is an informed choice: a decision based on the best information available and not influenced by faulty beliefs or intense feelings. The best choice has the highest probability of reward with the lowest risk of an unpleasant outcome. When you are aware of the danger of reacting foolhardily to an intense feeling, pausing to reflect on your choices and their consequences will give you control of yourself, the emotion, and, most likely, the situation.

CONTROLLING DESIRE

Temptation is everywhere. Most social activities are centered on food and drink. Many family events are feasts. Movie theaters and sports arenas offer every unhealthy "treat" imaginable. Then there is the temptation to skip exercising in favor of something more appealing—at least in the moment. The desire to have something that isn't needed or affordable and the urge to speak unkindly about someone are other examples of the ways we are tempted to do something that likely will be regretted later. Resisting the temptation to do something you might regret is an internal struggle between immediate and future gratification and between an urge and self-control.

The desire for immediate gratification is a challenge for most of us. It can be a curse for someone with diabetes. Winning the struggle between desire and self-restraint is at the core of being emotionally smart.

Certainly, the best and often easiest way to resist temptation is to not put yourself in its path. At a picnic where the desserts are on the table at your left and the salads and veggies are to the right, staying away from the table to the left would reduce the risk of giving way to temptation. Chapter 12 presents a strategy intended to "anticipate and eliminate" situations that might be undesirable or even harmful. If you expect most of the offerings will be unacceptable, before going to that picnic, prepare and take your own healthy treats. Staying away from temptation is a good strategy, but there are many circumstances that provoke unfavorable urges that are unavoidable.

> *Sally is making a strong effort to better manage her blood glucose levels. She has a weakness for chocolate and has made a commitment to allow herself a small amount of the sweet treat once a month. She is in the fourth month of her goal when she is faced with an incredibly delicious-looking and rich chocolate cake. She is at a friend's birthday party, and it is on the table right there in her face. The urge to have a piece of the cake is strong, bordering on craving it. The voice in her head says, "Oh, go ahead and have it. You can get back to your commitment tomorrow." Or she might think, "Hey, I've kept to the vow for over 3 months, which is remarkable. I deserve a treat." The seeker of instant gratification always has a way of rationalizing his or her behavior.*

In this instance, Sally knows she will regret eating the cake, and she is trying to resolve the struggle by arguing that she deserves it. The challenge is to find a frame that makes resisting eating the cake a reward rather than feeling deprived or punished. Sally has to give the act of delaying pleasure a positive meaning. She starts with the **mindful question**:

MQ | *How can I reframe this situation to do the right thing and feel good about it?*

Mindfully engaged in self-talk (reflection), Sally is able to override the urge to do what her objective self does not want to do. Her answer is, "If I eat that, I know I will be sorry, and I will not like myself for giving in. And I know, too, that if I turn away from the temptation, 10 minutes from now, I will forget it with no regrets. Most of all, I will feel good about myself because I was able to exercise good self-control." Initially, Sally's frame was, "I am a child who is being deprived and my only choice is to have a tantrum." Her reframe is, "I can make the right choice and take good care of myself. I will reward myself later on for exercising good control."

When resisting immediate gratification has a positive meaning, it not only overrides the undesirable urge and eliminates feelings of deprivation and self-pity, it also builds confidence, pride, and self-esteem.

EMPATHIC ACCEPTANCE

So far, the focus has been on "I" feelings—emotions you are feeling. Empathic acceptance is about the feelings of those with whom you interact and who are expressing their emotions. In "transcending emotional stressors" or "controlling desire," you are the subject of the emotions; you are the one feeling them. In this case, you are the object of someone else's feelings.

In the pie-and-hostess scenario, you were the one being pressured to eat the pie. Now, look at the same situation from a different perspective—from the other person's state of mind. Imagine this person holding the pie up to your mouth and insisting that you have to eat it. She is being obnoxious, and you are losing patience. Although you probably do not know the frame that is driving her behavior, it is clear that it is a faulty one. There are two possible explanations for this forceful action: either she is a vicious person with malicious intent or she really believes that she is acting in your best interest. Given that there is no reason to believe that she wants to do harm, it is reasonable to accept that her behavior is based on a belief or beliefs that are misguided. From this perspective, it is in your and her best interests to respond to the onslaught with empathy, with gracious understanding of her behavior. From an empathic perspective, you do not become emotionally involved and thereby risk escalating an already unpleasant situation. Furthermore, it opens the possibility of a meaningful dialogue. Consider these *mindful questions*:

MQ	*How can I turn this situation around for both of us?*
	How can I help her feel OK without having to eat the pie?

One possible response is, "I know you mean well, but insisting that I eat what I do not want is not helpful. I have diabetes, and eating the pie is not in my plan today. How about joining me for tea or coffee, and we can talk about diabetes?" One of the frustrations I hear from people with diabetes stems from the interaction of others who, at best, have only a shallow understanding of the disease. Not being informed or being misinformed about diabetes, they come across as judgmental or not approving of something that they do not understand. With the invitation to get to know each other better, you have the opportunity to educate the other person about your condition and its many aspects.

Whenever you are being unjustly criticized or worse, understand that the one who is acting with hostility is operating from his or her belief system, which is obviously misguided. You have several choices. You can try to defend yourself, which is senseless because the charge against you is groundless anyway. You can counterattack, which is just as senseless and would have an unfavorable outcome. You can react with empathy, which is responding to the reality of the situation rather than expanding on some misunderstanding or misbelief. Accepting someone's objectionable behavior with compassion is not easy, but if the relationship is worth keeping, it is a good way to go.

What Are Some Common Causes of Maladaptive Reactions to Feelings?

Some of us are prone to maladaptive reactions to our emotions. Many factors can determine one's tendency to act one way or another. To some extent, we inherit patterns of thinking and behaving. Although there may be a biological link, a bias to an emotion and the reaction to it are likely to have been influenced by lessons learned in childhood.

The trials and tribulations of early life are recorded in conscious and unconscious memory and play out throughout life. Children who have had experiences that diminish their self-concept and self-esteem—such as rejection, abandonment, and abuse—are prone to be emotionally sensitive and tend to react to their feelings ineffectively. Early traumas can be especially troublesome as they become strongly imprinted in the brain's emotional system. Subsequently, another condition that has some resemblance to the original traumas arouses both the memory and the corresponding feelings as if what has just happened is a repeat of the trauma. Cultural factors can also have an effect on an individual's emotional disposition. Expressing feelings more intensely, with more passion, is more common in some parts of the world than others.

A pattern of troublesome emotional behavior may be a sign of a disturbance that needs professional assistance. The person who often feels sad, angry, or inadequate or who is always anxious or who strongly craves something that is not healthy would do well to consult a professional mental health counselor for an evaluation.

What Are the Barriers to Being Emotionally Smart?

Make a commitment to being emotionally smart and practice the principles and skills in this chapter and in all of Part 3, especially Chapters 8 (Reframing), 11 (Problem Solving), and 12 (Anticipate It). Keep to your commitment, and you can overcome any barriers.

With few exceptions, acting mindlessly on how you feel gives power to the emotion and disregards thoughtful control of what is causing the feeling. Being emotionally smart gives you the power and control needed for keeping your emotions and the emotions of others from getting in the way of the efforts to manage your diabetes.

Just as you may be challenged frequently to reframe faulty beliefs, you may also be challenged to control your reaction to your emotions. When you reframe a belief, you change what it means to you and what it does to you. When you take charge of how you react to a feeling, you choose what the emotion does to you. You are in control. Your brain is programmed to react physically and emotionally to a wide range of stimuli, but the program in your brain may not be working in your best interest. Taking control of how you think and act—despite how you feel—gives you the power and the ability to manage the stress of diabetes and other hardships.

CHAPTER 6

Essential People Skills

Having good people skills can be a key to success. Conversely, having poor people skills is an invitation for strife and stress. Even the most independent individual has to relate to and even depend on others. The quality of relationships often depends on using core people skills: the ability to communicate effectively, to be appropriately assertive, and to be able to resolve conflicts constructively.

A common frustration for people with diabetes is interacting with others—family, friends, care providers, medical insurance representatives, bosses, and coworkers—about diabetes-related matters. Having good people skills facilitates constructive interactions and, thus, avoids unnecessary frustration and distress. Effective people skills are essential to the objective of minimizing stress and its negative effects on both diabetes management and quality of life.

Why Are the Essential People Skills So Important?

You interact with someone for a reason. It may be to get something or to give or not give something. The process of communicating a point of view, a need, or a desire can be very complicated because it involves the belief systems of everyone involved as well as their ability to effectively send and receive information. When the stakes are high and the outcome of the interaction is important, using core skills can make the difference between success and failure.

The essential people skills give you the power to send and receive messages with the assurance that they will be clear and the intent unmistakable. These skills give you the ability to stand up for yourself when your needs and rights are being disregarded, and they provide the capability to negotiate a positive outcome in a situation where there are conflicting positions that might result in a negative outcome.

These skills, individually and combined, have a domino effect of positives. When someone is being disrespectful and you stand up for yourself, your self-esteem gets a boost. Furthermore, you avoid feeling resentful or feeling inadequate for not being assertive on your own behalf. Being able to communicate your needs clearly and in a way that elicits the compassion of others builds self-confidence, and it is a way for developing a comforting support network. Communicating well grows good relationships. Most importantly, the essential people skills prevent the onset or escalation of stress.

Will These Skills Help in Dealing with Diabetes?

People skills are important for dealing with diabetes because there are so many issues that involve or even depend on other people. You may have a general physician, endocrinologist, podiatrist, and nutritionist caring for you as well as their team of assistants. Have you ever been told something by a care provider that you didn't agree with or didn't understand, but you did not speak up? Have you avoided revealing something that concerned you because you were afraid your doctor would be displeased? Do you try to hide the fact that you have diabetes to avoid the possibility of being rejected? How many clashes have you had with family and friends that were caused by poor communications or none at all. The core people skills maximize your control of these stressors, which are common to diabetes and life in general.

Some individuals use good people skills in some situations, but are ineffectual in other circumstances. Some, for example, do well in communicating and asserting themselves in the workplace, but do poorly in a more intimate setting. Others may readily resolve conflicts at home, but fail at the office. The intent in this chapter is to prepare you to be skilled in every situation.

How Can I Develop These Skills?

COMMUNICATING EFFECTIVELY

Aside from idle conversation, the purpose in communicating with another is to produce an intentional reaction and to have a predetermined impact on the listener. The purpose may be simply to have the receiver understand the message; or it might be more complex, like trying to persuade someone to change an opinion. Whatever the intention, it is essential to get your message across with absolute clarity.

As the receiver of a message, the primary objective is to understand the exact meaning of what was said. There are specific techniques for giving and receiving a message.

Getting Your Message Across

This objective involves several strategies:

1. *Be mindful of what you want to say.* When the stakes are high, writing down your message beforehand will give you the opportunity to review and sharpen your presentation.

2. *Say exactly what you mean, and say it kindly and honestly.* Expressing yourself kindly does not mean stifling your feelings; it means avoiding expressing feelings in a hostile manner, which would only work against you.

3. *Stay focused and avoid distractions.* Do not let reactions to your message draw you away from your agenda.

4. *If there is any doubt that your message was understood, ask the other person to repeat what you said.* Even if there is no doubt, it is wise to ask for the repetition of what you said, especially when a misunderstanding could have serious consequences.

5. *If emotion is a part of your message, level with the person with whom you are communicating.* Calmly and clearly express what you are feeling. There is a difference between saying, "I'm so angry I could scream" and actually screaming. Yelling won't get you what you want.

6. *Ask for feedback.* Ask if the receiver of your message understands it. Ask if he or she has any questions about what has been said. Questions like, "You look perplexed; is there a problem with what I said?" or simply, "What is your reaction to this?" can help clarify and eliminate any barriers to resolving the conflict.

7. *Do not assume anything.* Know whether there is agreement or disagreement on the issue raised. If there is disagreement, consider negotiating a satisfactory outcome (see Resolving Conflict Effectively on page 119).

8. *If there is a disagreement, still validate the other's position.* This does not mean you agree with what is being said, but it does mean you respect the right of the other person to have a different viewpoint.

9. *Watch for facial expressions or a tone of voice that may indicate a nonverbal reaction to the message.* If you think what you have seen is relevant, share your observation with the other person.

10. *Pay attention to the body language of the person with whom you are talking.* If the other person seems uncomfortable, ask if your perception is correct; and if it is, ascertain what is causing the uneasiness.

Getting the Message

Effective communication is an interactive process between the sender and receiver of a message. Getting the message also requires a set of skills.

1. *Listen keenly to what is being said.* Stay with the message being sent; then take time to collect your thoughts before you respond. Resist thinking about your response until the sender has finished talking.

2. *Be committed to getting the message.* As the receiver, your purpose is to fully grasp the intent of the sender.

3. *Stay focused and avoid distractions.* Making assumptions about the sender's intent or allowing your attention to drift is not in your or the sender's best interests.

4. *Be open-minded without prejudging the message.* Nothing good can happen if you evaluate the message before it is fully communicated.

5. *Ask for clarification when you are not certain about what has been said.* If there is any uncertainty about what you have heard, ask for the message to be repeated. If you are confused, ask that the message be stated in a different way, which should help make the communication understandable.

6. *State in your own words what you believe was said.* Give the sender feedback. Start with "Did you say . . . ?" or "Did I understand you to mean . . . ?"

7. *Do not assume anything.* Being clear about what has been said and making certain that your reaction is clear to the sender is necessary. It does not matter how many times the sender and receiver communicate back and forth to achieve clarity; being clear is what matters.

8. *Level with the sender about your reactions and feelings regarding what is being said.* It is important to express how you feel in a nonthreatening manner.

9. *If you disagree with any part of the message, let the sender know clearly what the problem is for you.* Express your disagreement with empathy (see Chapter 5) and with respect for the viewpoint of the sender. Be kind and honest, and you will do well.

Avoid Pitfalls

The more mindful you are of the barriers to communicating effectively, the less likely you are to suffer from them. Here are some of the common obstacles to avoid.

1. *Perceiving the interaction as a contest.* You will not send a clear and honest message if you start with the belief that you have to win and the other has to lose. You will not hear the message if you are competing with the sender, thinking how you can win, or how you can disprove the sender's viewpoint or top it. The need to be right regardless of the facts is a sure loser.

2. *Thinking about what you will say about the message before it has been fully communicated.* If you want to prepare your response, you can do it after the message has been completed. There is nothing wrong with pausing to think about the matter being discussed. There is nothing wrong with saying, "I need time to think about what you said."

3. *Listening selectively to what is being said.* If, for example, your frame for the sender is that he only wants something from you, then you might only hear the part of the message that fits with your expectations. While it might be true that the sender wants something, it may also be a worthwhile request, but you won't hear that part of the communication.

4. *Making assumptions about what the sender has in mind or how the receiver will react.* You are not a mind reader and assuming that you already know what is being said closes your mind to what is really being communicated. Listening with keen interest can avoid undue hardship.

5. *Being the fixer, even when you're not asked to be.* There are times when the messenger simply wants to be heard, perhaps to vent a frustration, and is not expecting the listener to fix anything. Trying to fix something that you do not have the power to repair can be very frustrating to all concerned.

6. *Needing to please.* Saying "yes" when you really want to say "no" may please the messenger in the short term, but it is likely to be unpleasant for both parties in the long run.

7. *Escalating emotions.* When the message or the response to it is emotionally charged, the goal of all concerned is to be emotionally smart. If the emotional level is intense, a good strategy is for one of the participants to call a time-out (see Chapter 5).

An important part of learning a new skill is to evaluate how you are doing. These *mindful questions* will help you to assess your progress:

MQ	*Did I send or receive the message effectively?*
	What evidence is there that what was intended to happen did take place?
	If the message was not sent or received clearly, what could I have done differently that would have worked?
	What have I learned from this experience?

For examples of effective communications, see People Skills in Action—Communicating Effectively on pages 114–115.

BEING EFFECTIVELY ASSERTIVE

Being able to stand up for yourself and to defend your personal rights, including setting boundaries with others, is important to living well and avoiding unnecessary stress in relationships. There are times when being assertive is essential for achieving a successful outcome. However, there are personal beliefs that keep people from expressing their feelings ("Whatever I do, you will think I am stupid") or keep them from preventing others from taking advantage of them ("If I say no, I will be the subject of endless wrath").

The Range of Assertive Behaviors

A common barrier to being assertive is misunderstanding the distinctions among assertiveness, aggressiveness, and hostility. Many individuals believe that all acts of assertiveness are the same and therefore inappropriate, if not dangerous. It will be helpful to think of assertive behavior on a continuum from passive to hostile:

Passive $\longrightarrow$ Assertive $\longrightarrow$ Aggressive $\longrightarrow$ Hostile

Passive behavior is basically the absence of assertiveness. Passive individuals say "yes" or "fine" when they do not mean it. They apologize and justify themselves excessively and are unable to protect themselves from the unreasonable demands of others.

PEOPLE SKILLS IN ACTION— COMMUNICATING EFFECTIVELY

Jessie has had episodes of extreme low blood glucose levels when she was unable to effectively respond to her condition. Acting to prevent a serious problem at work, she asked a coworker, Polly, to be her support person. Jessie informed Polly about hypoglycemia and the symptoms she experiences in that state. She asked Polly to be aware of the signs that her glucose level was low. Jessie was thoughtful and precise in her descriptions and in telling Polly what to do.

Jessie: *I know I have given you a lot to take in. If you would like, I'll give you some printed material that should help. But for now, how about repeating back to me the signals that indicate my blood glucose level has dropped to a dangerous level? And what would you do?*

Jessie has done a good job sending her message to Polly, and her coworker was able to repeat in detail what she was told. Of course, this was a compliment to Polly, too, who had listened to Jessie's message carefully. In this matter, a miscommunication could have serious consequences.

Jessie: *Wow, you got it all, but you seem to be uneasy. Are you concerned about doing this?*

Polly: *Well, I have to admit that it is a little scary. What if I don't do it right?*

Although Polly didn't verbalize her concern, Jessie heard it in her voice and made it an issue. She did not assume that Polly was OK with it just because she had not directly expressed any concern. In turn, Polly was able to reveal that she was feeling uneasy anticipating the possibility of being responsible for her coworker's well-being.

Jessie: *The last thing I would want is to make you uncomfortable. I intend to do everything I can to prevent having an extreme low blood glucose episode, but knowing that I have someone nearby to help me if it happens is so comforting. I'm sure it would not be fun for you, but I am certain that you would do just fine. And remember, if the episode was severe, you should call 911, which is what you would do for any emergency.*

Polly sent the message that she needed some assurance that she was capable of doing what would be needed if Jessie's blood glucose level dropped substantially. Jessie understood the intent of the message and gave Polly the response she needed.

Polly: *I appreciate your confidence in me. I hope it never happens, but I will do my best if it is needed. And I would like to see the printed material you mentioned. The more I know, the more confident I will feel.*

By communicating effectively, both Jessie and Polly were able to have the intent of their messages satisfied.

Assertive people are honest and direct about their thoughts, needs, and feelings. They do not tolerate a violation of their basic rights or boundaries. Those who assert themselves appropriately are confident and secure "in their own skin."

Being aggressive is being more forceful when assertive behavior is not respected. If, for example, you told a friend that you did not want her to inform others in a social situation that you have diabetes and she kept doing it, then an aggressive approach would be to tell her that you will stop going to places with her if she does not honor your request. If she continued to talk about your diabetes in social settings, then the next level of aggressiveness might be to end the relationship. Being aggressive does not violate the rights of another; it is an escalation of firmness for your own well-being without doing harm to someone.

Hostile behavior is overly aggressive. It is disrespecting the rights and well-being of another. In the case of the so-called friend who insists on telling everyone you have diabetes, the hostile individual might verbally attack or, at worse, shove the person who continues to disregard the appeal to stop broadcasting your diabetes. Of course, extreme hostile behavior can escalate to physically harming someone. Hostile behavior is only appropriate in defending oneself from physical harm.

Assertive behavior is necessary and essential for taking the best care of yourself. The process for being assertive involves several mindful actions:

- Make a commitment to acting assertively as an essential part of your self-care.
- Identify and eliminate any barriers you have to acting assertively (see the *mindful questions* after this list).
- Be mindful of situations that have or could lead you to passive or hostile behavior.
- In any situation in which you are not being appropriately assertive, ask these *mindful questions*:

MQ

Do I have a right to be assertive? Are my rights and values being ignored or violated?

What frame or frames (beliefs) are keeping me from asserting myself and from declaring my rights?

Am I being held back by one of these faulty frames: "I don't deserve it," "I don't want to offend anyone," or "I'm afraid of being rejected?" Is some other faulty frame stopping me?

What frame is causing me to be overly assertive or inappropriately aggressive?

What frame will enable me to assert myself in this situation?

For the last question, try this frame: "I have a right to stand up for myself. It is important to be respected. I deserve it!"

Setting Boundaries

We use locks on doors and walls or fences to separate our property from other properties. They serve to keep out what we do not want in. Similarly, it is important to establish boundaries in relationships. A boundary can be stated in terms of proximity, that is, by how close you are willing to have someone get to you. It can be in terms of familiarity—the degree to which private matters are shared. A boundary declares your right to keep a part of yourself to yourself. Boundaries with others vary with the level of the relationship. The more trustworthy the association, the fewer the boundaries; but even in the closest relationship, some limits may be desirable. Not being able to declare your boundaries with family, friends, coworkers, and others who are significant to your life can be very stressful. Not setting limits invites intrusive and, perhaps, even abusive behavior. Setting boundaries is essential to healthy self-care.

Barriers to Being Assertive in Setting Boundaries

Being aware of what keeps you from standing up for yourself is the first step in eliminating the barrier to being appropriately assertive. Generally, a lack of assertive behavior is associated with the belief that one does not have the right to act on one's own behalf. Like the origin of most faulty beliefs, the idea that one does not have the right to his or her thoughts, feelings, and needs usually originates in childhood, when the actions of authority figures may be perceived as proof that one does not deserve better. With this foundation, the child grows up lacking confidence and self-esteem and becomes overly dependent on others. With this background, the individual is unable to be effectively assertive and is compelled to please others, at great personal cost.

Being assertive can be risky. Standing up for yourself may not be appreciated by the person you are standing up to. Many of the frames that oppose being assertive are rooted in the fear of being disliked or, worse, being rejected.

Here are some frames that impair assertive behavior:
- "I don't deserve better."
- "Asking for anything for myself will get me in trouble."
- "Standing up for myself is disrespectful of others."
- "Setting boundaries is being selfish."
- "It is weak to want or need anything from someone."
- "Those in authority are always right."

Each of these frames needs to be replaced.

When it is difficult to assert yourself, to demand the regard and respect of another, consider these *mindful questions*:

MQ | *What frame is keeping me from asserting myself in this situation?*

Is what I am feeling caused by a faulty, irrational frame?

What frame will enable me to stand up for myself despite any uncomfortable feelings?

Do I need to set a boundary? Am I reluctant to do it? Why?

Generally, frames have matching feelings and actions. If the frame for being assertive is threatening, you will feel afraid and avoid the encounter. Choosing a frame that contests the fear can be effective. Here is an example: "I feel scared because I am meeting with an endocrinologist for the first time, and I was told that he can be feisty with his patients. The feeling is real; the reason is not. I am more than the feeling. I will assert myself and whatever happens, I can handle it." This frame is positive, it is rational, and it instills the confidence to act. See People Skills in Action—Being Assertive (pages 120–121) for more examples of being assertive.

RESOLVING CONFLICT EFFECTIVELY

Disagreements between two or more individuals occur often. The dispute may have to do with what to fix for supper or what movie to see, or the disagreement can be serious. A conflict is a disagreement for which the stakes are higher. For our purposes, a conflict is the perception by one or more of the involved parties that their needs or interests are in jeopardy. The greater the value of the need or interest, the more intense the conflict will be. Conflicts can be psychologically, physically, and materially costly; therefore, resolving a conflict is necessary, and the sooner the better.

A conflict can be quite complex; it can be intense and highly emotional. Two or more individuals in conflict involve multiple belief systems, values, temperaments, and levels of knowledge about the issues involved in the dispute. Furthermore, how each person perceives the other parties to the disagreement can make the negotiations more difficult. If, for example, you are trying to end a conflict and you perceive the other party as an authority figure with a lot of power, that perception is likely to have a significant impact on how well you do on your own behalf. Having a solid foundation for resolving conflicts is a powerful equalizer.

PEOPLE SKILLS IN ACTION— BEING ASSERTIVE

Harris has been unable to meet his diabetes goals. His blood glucose levels tend to be above 250 mg/dL. His family physician treats him. Harris has an appointment with the doctor every 3 months, at which time adjustments are made to his medications based on routine bloodwork. Not feeling well most of the time, he is frustrated, but he has also been reluctant to share this with his doctor. Harris does everything he can to avoid disapproval. However, at the most recent appointment, Harris questions the treatment plan.

Harris: *Dr. Keller, my treatment is not going well. Is there something else I can be doing to better manage my diabetes?*

Motivated by his frustration, Harris is able to change his passivity-driven frame from "disapproval is dangerous and to be avoided at any price" to the self-respecting frame, "I deserve better, and I have a right to stand up for myself."

Dr. Keller: *I'm doing everything there is to do to help you. I can't follow you everywhere and watch what you do, so I don't know what the problem is. If you don't do what I tell you to do, then you can't blame me.*

The doctor's reaction is defensive and hostile. He believes Harris is questioning his competence, and he responds by accusing his patient of being at fault by not complying with his instructions.

Harris: *You have been very helpful. I would be a lot worse off if it wasn't for you. I just thought there might be something new I could try to get better control of my blood glucose levels.*

The doctor's hostile manner has scared Harris, and he is backing down. His belief that "disapproval is dangerous" has been revived, and he is momentarily unable to hold his ground.

Harris: *I have been attending a diabetes support group, and everyone there is treated by an endocrinologist.*

Still intimidated by his doctor's displeasure, Harris is not able to directly state his desire to see a diabetes specialist. Instead, he put the onus on members of the support group—if anyone is at fault for this idea, it is not him.

Dr. Keller: *Well, they don't know what they are talking about. I have treated hundreds of patients with diabetes, and no one else has ever complained. If you would do what I tell you to do, you would not be having so much trouble. You don't need to see another doctor; you just need to get your act together and take my advice seriously.*

The doctor continues to be defensive and critical of Harris.

Harris: *I haven't done everything I should every time, but I think I have been trying hard to manage my diabetes. If your only response is to insult me, then I can't trust that you are acting in my best interest. I have decided to see someone else to treat my diabetes.*

Using his discomfort as a signal, Harris was able to reflect more on what was keeping him from asserting himself. He became aware that he was reacting, too, to the belief that authority figures are always right and to oppose them was not safe. He recognized an old pattern of perceiving authority figures as having all of the power, which meant he had none. The absurdity of this belief almost made him laugh. And, finally, he was able to express his absolute right to stand up for himself.

Fundamentals for Resolving Conflict

Understanding these basics is essential to being successful in resolving disagreements at any level of intensity.

- The best approach to resolving a conflict is to find a win-win solution. A conflict is not a contest in which there has to be a winner and a loser. Certainly, there are situations for which it is not possible for both parties to win, at least not completely. However, each party must get something meaningful from the agreed-upon resolution.

- Forming an alliance—an association with all parties in the conflict—that is based on advancing common interests increases the probability of achieving a win-win outcome.

- In presenting your position, mindfully consider the costs and benefits it will impose on the other side. Understanding the position of the other increases the likelihood of forming a collaborative effort.

- The process for conflict resolution is a give-and-take, back-and-forth endeavor. It almost always requires compromise. Winning rarely means getting everything you want.

- Conflicts are often emotionally charged, but the process of ending the disagreement requires earnest control of feelings. The more intense the negotiations, the more important it is to be "emotionally smart." Few things can be more disruptive to the process of conflict resolution than unrestrained emotions.

- Each party to a conflict has needs, interests, and an agenda. Understanding these will be helpful in generating a positive outcome. It is as important to understand the issues of the other parties in a dispute as it is to know your own concerns.

- An open mind is essential. The ability to see all sides of a disagreement—to respect viewpoints that differ from your own—encourages a collaborative effort.

- The resolution of a conflict often requires the techniques of problem solving, including brainstorming for possible solutions (see Chapter 11).

- In agreeing on a solution to a conflict, mindfully consider the costs and benefits of your decision.
- And before the final handshake, make certain that all parties have the same understanding of the agreement. Use the communication skills presented earlier in this chapter to be sure that everyone has heard and agreed to the same conditions.

Styles for Resolving Conflict

Some individuals are locked into one style of conflict resolution; they see only one way to approach a conflict, which is very limiting. You will be most effective when you are able to use the approach that best suits the situation. It can also be to your advantage to recognize the style that is being used by the other party in the conflict.

- *Avoidance.* Some individuals react to conflict by avoiding dealing with it. Although it may be of value to delay addressing a conflict to seek more information or advice, avoiding dealing with a conflict is likely to make matters worse. Avoidance is practiced for several reasons: a lack of interest, a lack of confidence, or a fear of what might happen if the matter is addressed.
- *Accommodation.* People who use this style tend to submit to the needs of others. They may be motivated by a need to avoid offending people or by the belief that they cannot win, so giving in is the best choice. Certainly, being accommodating is appropriate when what has been proposed is beneficial.
- *Competition.* This style is aggressive and confrontational. Individuals who use this approach are not concerned about the reactions of others. They will try to control the situation with their intimidating manner. In some circumstances, confrontation is necessary, but being continuously competitive will make matters worse more often than not. This style is likely to prohibit a collaborative effort to achieve a win-win resolution.

- *Compromise.* This style requires all parties to have reasonably similar agendas. The issue in question may not be that important, so there is a willingness to resolve the matter quickly, or compromise may be the best or only choice to make. With this approach, there is a series of tradeoffs for which the costs and benefits are fair to all concerned.
- *Collaborate.* When the stakes are high and the relationship between the participants is trusting, the willingness to collaborate can be strong. Individuals who do not perceive themselves as having a considerable advantage in the negotiations might also be motivated to work together. With this approach, the parties' interests and efforts are synchronized to realize the same goal. This is the most likely style to achieve a win-win outcome.
- *Disengage.* There are times when a conflict cannot be resolved and there is no other choice but to disengage and to have the parties agree to disagree. This step should be the last recourse. It should be used only if every possibility has been exhausted.

Each style has its place in resolving conflicts. Certainly collaboration is the style of choice so long as all parties to the problem are genuinely motivated to work together in a reciprocal manner.

Steps for Resolving Conflict

When the costs of failing or the benefits of succeeding are high or when the disagreement is complex, it can be helpful to use a structured approach to addressing the conflict. Here is a process for undoing a conflict and for turning a disagreement into a mutually agreeable understanding.

1. *Prepare.* Do your homework. Identify as clearly as possible the issues that are involved on all sides. Use the fundamentals of conflict resolution (see Styles for Resolving Conflict on pages 123–124) and avoid

the barriers to a successful outcome (see Barriers to Resolving Conflict on pages 126–129).

2. *Use the communication skills described at the beginning of this chapter to facilitate a meaningful discussion and constructive negotiations.*

3. *Establish mutually agreeable ground rules.* Predetermined behavioral boundaries may be necessary to prevent highly charged emotions from disrupting the process. To this end, it may be useful to have the parties agree to honor anyone's request for a timeout if emotions get intense. This means that if anyone asks for a timeout, the negotiations will stop for a specific and reasonable period of time. After cooling down during the timeout, negotiations are resumed.

4. *When possible, develop an alliance with your adversary.* Seek to establish a collaborative mood built on mutual interests, trust, and a win-win attitude.

5. *Jointly identify the disagreement, preferably in terms of interests and needs.* If the conflict is complex, divide the problem into smaller, workable parts.

6. *Keep the effort focused on the matters mutually agreed upon, avoiding wasteful distractions.*

7. *Use the principles of sound problem solving (Chapter 11).* Focus on solutions, not the problem.

8. *Encourage everyone to offer solutions to the conflict.* If necessary, use brainstorming to generate alternative solutions (see pages 190–191).

9. *With a give-and-take, back-and-forth attitude, negotiate a solution to the conflict that is mutually agreeable.*

10. *If agreement cannot be reached, schedule another meeting, challenging the other to commit to finding a satisfactory solution to the conflict.* In preparing for the follow-up meeting, try to identify what prevented the process from working before.

Barriers to Resolving Conflict

For every party involved in trying to end a conflict, there are several factors that can get in the way of reaching an agreement. Being mindful of potential obstacles increases the chance of avoiding or overcoming them. Here are some common barriers to bringing a conflict to a satisfactory conclusion.

- *Poor communications.* When you fail to convey your message with unmistakable clarity, you have jeopardized your chance of accomplishing your objective. And when you do not listen intently to what is being presented, you won't "see" the other's point of view. You likely will miss opportunities to move the negotiations forward. Or worse, you might wrongly agree to something because you misunderstood the terms of the agreement.

- *"I'm right; you're wrong."* In my role as a mental health counselor, one of my favorite questions has been, "Would you rather be right or happy?" Having counseled many couples, I rarely have seen a relationship in which one party was right and the other was wrong. Most often, the positions of both had some degree of correctness as well as some measure of wrongness. The problem was that each only paid attention to what was right for him or her. Believing that your way of looking at the conflict is the "right" way and that anyone else's viewpoint is "wrong" will make reaching an agreement difficult, if not impossible.

- *Hidden agendas.* Nothing can block resolving a conflict more than a hidden agenda. If you are trying to settle a disagreement with someone and you or the other person has an unstated agenda that opposes what has been stated, the end result of your attempt to reach an agreement will be frustration and despair. For example, negotiating with an insurance company about medical treatment can be frustrating because the insurer has an agenda about the cost of the care, an agenda that is not stated but may affect the outcome.

Andrew and Joan have been discussing possible destinations for a vacation together without success. Every suggestion has not been acceptable to Joan, and Andrew is becoming increasingly annoyed. The problem is that Joan does not want to go away with Andrew, but she does not want to hurt her friend's feelings. Her hidden agenda makes a resolution impossible; instead it is creating stress for both of them.

- *The illusion of control.* The fear of losing control is a common barrier to many endeavors.

  Jordan often acts in opposition to the advice of his wife and his physician because he does not want anyone to control his life. His blood glucose levels are consistently high. Jordan believes that not doing what anyone else wants him to do means he is in control, but he is steadfastly spinning out of control.

  Acting on the illusion of control will produce more chaos than order.

- *Name calling.* Emotions can run high in the process of negotiating an end to a conflict, especially when a participant is frightened or offended by an aspect of the proposed agreement. The person feeling threatened may counter by verbally attacking the other party. Believing the negotiations are going the wrong way, he or she might call the counterpart selfish, controlling, devious, or worse. This scenario blocks any reasonable solution to the conflict. Instead, an escalation of animosity and distrust is likely. Anger can be expressed appropriately: "I believe that you aren't listening to my issues, which is very frustrating." Similarly, the response to anger can be constructive: "I am sorry you are so upset. Help me to understand why." Calling someone a derogatory name is acting out the feeling. While it might feel good at the moment, the end result is likely to be self-defeating.

- *Polarizing.* Thinking at the extremes makes resolving a difference difficult, if not impossible. Thinking everything is right or wrong, black or white, or good or bad opposes one of the most important needs for effective conflict resolution: flexibility. The lack of flexibility narrows the options for ending a disagreement. Being resilient is essential to the give-and-take, back-and-forth process that is essential to negotiating a good-natured outcome.
- *Kitchen sinking.* This term has been used to describe individuals who will throw anything into an argument to win. The image of throwing in the kitchen sink emphasizes the absurdity of this style.

> *Joy wants her husband to agree to changes in their eating style. She wants them to eat out less often and to have more salads and less pasta for dinner. What he hears is "only salads and no pasta," which is totally unacceptable to him. Instead of expressing his concerns, which would have given Joy the chance to make her intention clear, he blocked the possibility of a positive outcome by throwing everything but the kitchen sink into the disagreement. When Joy suggested that eating at home would be less costly than going to restaurants, he said they could save more if she didn't spend so much on clothes, makeup, and the hairdresser. On the matter of salad versus pasta, he said it was all about her need to control him, to always have it her way, and noted several completely unrelated examples of his contention.*

- *Door slamming.* When the reaction to a sincere effort to resolve a conflict is disregarded or the response is dismissive or unrelated to the matter at hand, the door has been slammed. The person who responds in this manner does not want to deal with the problem.

> *Rose wants her husband to be more supportive, to show an interest in what she does to manage her diabetes, and, perhaps, to even remind her to*

take her medications. Each time she tries to start a conversation about her wishes, her husband says, "There you go again." The door has been slammed. She walks away in a huff.

The challenge for Rose is to do something that keeps the door from shutting in her face. The **mindful questions** are:

MQ | *His behavior is so frustrating, but walking away doesn't help. How can I reframe my reaction to keep the discussion from stalling?*

What about my requests are causing him to slam the door on what I am asking for?

How can I present my needs so they do not threaten or otherwise disengage him?

Resolving a conflict begins with pausing and using **mindful questions** to reflect on what choices you have to fix undesirable circumstances. Calm reflection, followed by a choice independent of emotions, is claiming your true power. It is the way to minimize, if not prevent, undue stress when conflict occurs.

The conflict between Janine and Edie in the box below was both unpleasant and unhealthy for both of them. The levels of stress were high. Janine's frustration and Edie's fear were constantly provoked. By using good people skills, Janine was able to negotiate an agreement that worked for both of them. She used the give-and-take approach effectively. Both of them had to make compromises that made a win-win solution possible. The ability to communicate, to be assertive, and to resolve conflicts is essential to successfully interacting with others. Each skill can be a vital tool for achieving the best possible management of your diabetes.

PEOPLE SKILLS IN ACTION— RESOLVING CONFLICT

This interaction between Janine, a 24-year-old who has type 1 diabetes, and her mother, Edie, demonstrates the use of each of the core people skills for ending a conflict.

Janine: *Mom, I need you to stop hovering over me and questioning me and telling me what to do. I can take care of myself. I know I have made some mistakes in the past, but I have learned how to avoid letting my blood glucose level get too low.*

The initial message is simple and clear, but raising the issue of her mistakes may unnecessarily complicate the conversation. Janine may have assumed that her mother would raise the matter, which may be correct, but why invite it?

Edie: *Honey, having to call the paramedics is very serious. I worry that you will let your blood glucose level drop again, and there may not be someone there to help you.*

Edie has picked up on Janine's reference to her mistakes. She is responding as if it is a contest to win—that is, to prove to her daughter that she has to continue to hover over her and direct her diabetes care.

Janine: *I know those episodes scared you, and I am sorry, but they were months ago, and I know better. I really need you to trust that I can take care of myself.*

Janine has done well by validating her mother's anxiety. It would have been a mistake to tell her mother that she shouldn't be concerned. Instead, Janine acknowledges her mother's discomfort and reiterates her readiness to take responsibility for herself. She raises the issue of trust, which is central for Janine.

Edie: *How can I trust you when I see you eating chocolate donuts? When you come home at 3:00 a.m. and I don't know where you have been all night? Trust you? When I get a call at work telling me you are in the emergency room?*

Edie heard Janine's reference to trust as accusing her of distrust. Edie reacts defensively by criticizing her daughter's past behavior. There is also a bit of kitchen sinking in her protest.

Janine: *I am not disagreeing with you about my past behavior. There were times when I did not act responsibly. I can't change what happened. All I ask is that we focus on the present and move on. I know what I have to do, and I know I can do it.*

I can't promise I will be perfect, but I am sure I won't have another extremely low blood glucose level that causes an emergency.

Janine is being realistic. She does not want to set it up so that any deviation in her behavior gives her mother cause to hover over her again.

Edie: *All I am doing is trying to help you manage your diabetes. I love you. It isn't easy to see my daughter suffer with this awful disease. Some nights I can't sleep at all, worrying if you are OK or not. When I can help you, I feel so much better. Put yourself in my place.*

Unfortunately, the reference to imperfection is taken as a warning of trouble rather than as a frank and reassuring statement. Reacting to her fear, Edie tries to make Janine feel guilty, implying that her daughter is not being sensitive to her motherly caring. She is determined to win, and her thinking is limited to an all-or-nothing perspective.

Janine: *This conversation is beginning to get to me. I am about to scream, so I think it would be smart to take a timeout. How about taking a 1-hour break? I'm going to check my blood glucose and then work out on the treadmill, which will help me think more clearly. Then, we can get together again and figure out something that works for both of us.*

Janine has wisely called a timeout. She is frustrated by her mother's inflexibility and her self-pitying tactic. Feeling the stress of the conflict, Janine is wise to check her blood glucose level.

(1 hour later . . .)

Edie: *Well, what brilliant idea did you come up with on the treadmill?*

She is aware of Janine's steadfastness, and her opening remark shows her displeasure. She is mocking her daughter's reference to thinking more clearly.

Janine: *Well, I do have an idea, and I hope you will like it. First, I am going to get a continuous glucose monitor, which will not only give me continual glucose readings but will signal when my blood glucose level changes by a preset amount or drops below a preset number. The device will be a huge help to me in guarding against extreme hypoglycemia. Second, I am going to keep a record of my blood glucose levels and what I eat, and I will give it to you each day. And if I am going to be out late, I will tell you where I am and keep my cell phone on in case you really need to* *call me. In return, I want you to agree to stop watching and questioning me and telling me what I should do. How about it?*

Taking the break worked. Janine was able to shift to a give-and-take approach, making a compromise to get some of what she wants and needs from her mother.

Edie: *Alright. Let's try it. You told me about the continuous glucose monitor, and I was hoping you would get it. I'll even pitch in half the cost.*

Pleased with the concessions offered to her, Edie offers one of her own: half the cost of the new continuous monitor.

Janine: *Great! And let's agree that we will have another meeting at the end of the month, which is almost 4 weeks from now, to see how we are doing with this plan.*

In planning a change, it is smart to follow up by evaluating whether the plan is working. Janine wisely makes the assessment a part of the agreement, which has the secondary benefit of assuring her mother that she will have the opportunity to express any problems she may have with the agreement.

CHAPTER 7

Choosing the Style in Lifestyle

What Is Lifestyle?

Everyone has a personal style, a collection of routines and patterns for daily life. Although one's lifestyle typically reflects an individual's attitudes, way of life, values, or world view, for many of us, a lifestyle develops mindlessly in response to events that occur and push or pull us one way or another. Decisions that lead to lifelong commitments, such as marriage and career, are often made on little information or reflection. Sometimes, the chosen pathways work out well. However, the choices may not always have the best possible outcome. A mindless approach is an invitation to missed opportunities as well as to stress and all of its misgivings.

Your lifestyle, the way you live your life, has several parts. Some aspects of lifestyle are obvious, including eating, sleeping, and exercising. Other important facets may not be as apparent or understood, such as being creative or frequent partying. This chapter will raise your awareness of the benefits of mindfully managing your lifestyle. By mindfully choosing the way you live your life, you are in control; you are in charge.

Why Is Lifestyle Important?

The more you are in control of your lifestyle, the better you can manage your diabetes and your overall well-being. The way you choose to live has a strong influence on how well you can manage your diabetes. Some aspects of lifestyle have a direct effect on diabetes management. How and what you eat and whether you exercise regularly make a big difference in your effort to maintain good glucose levels. Other aspects of lifestyle have a less direct, but considerable, impact on your ability to manage diabetes. Making happiness a deliberate part of your lifestyle is one example. Doing things that make you happy feels good, and the better you feel, the less likely you are to be unduly stressed.

Making mindless lifestyle choices can have dire results regarding diabetes management and your general well-being. Smoking, drinking excessively, and unchecked social media activity are lifestyle choices that are proven to have a serious negative impact on your health. Similarly, being hateful, being inflexible, or being judgmental bodes poorly for anyone who chooses to live in such a manner.

Choosing your lifestyle mindfully is enormously valuable. It eliminates the possibility of self-inflicted stress. By taking responsibility for your lifestyle, you are in control. Being in control enhances your confidence and self-esteem. Making conscious and purposeful decisions about the way you live will enrich every aspect of your life.

What Are the Basic Elements of a Healthy Lifestyle?

Some essential aspects of a healthy lifestyle are mindfulness (Chapter 3), letting go (Chapter 9), and humor (Chapter 13). This chapter presents the other vital ways of living well, starting with the basic elements.

BEING DIABETES SMART

Maximizing your power over diabetes requires being both stress smart and diabetes smart. Throughout this book, you will learn many ways to keep stress at a minimum, which is important for managing diabetes. Being diabetes smart means knowing everything about diabetes management and using that knowledge to keep your blood glucose levels in a healthy range.

It is essential to know the practical and technical aspects of glucose management, such as the interactions of carbohydrates and glucose, how to use a glucometer to check your blood glucose, how your medication acts on you over time, and how to deal with medical emergencies. Also, you need to know your body. Understanding how your blood glucose level changes with exercise and what symptoms you experience when your glucose level is too high or too low enables you to live well with diabetes.

Diabetes care is more than 90% self-care; the more you know, the better. Don't stop at Diabetes 101; get your self-directed master's degree. Many hospitals offer educational programs for individuals with diabetes. The Internet provides numerous resources. The American Diabetes Association website, www.diabetes.org, is an excellent resource. This website has many informative pages, including Diabetes Basics, which covers a wide range of information about management. The National Institute of Diabetes and Digestive and Kidney Diseases website, www.niddk.nih.gov, is another valuable resource. There are others, including the websites of JDRF (formerly known as the Juvenile Diabetes Research Foundation) (www.jdrf.org), the Centers for Disease Control and Prevention (www.cdc.gov/diabetes), the Joslin Diabetes Center (www.joslin.org), and the American Association of Diabetes Educators (diabeteseducator.org), to name a few (see Chapter 14: The Internet: Excellent with Caution for a thorough review of the World Wide Web as a resource for managing diabetes).

EATING SENSIBLY

Eating sensibly is essential to successful diabetes management, a subject you probably know a lot about. If not, there are numerous sources for learning about what to eat when you have diabetes: books, the Internet, and publications, such as the American Diabetes Association's magazine, *Diabetes Forecast*. Eating wisely is also about resisting the temptation to eat something when it is not in your best interest to do so (see Controlling Desire in Chapter 5). The focus in this chapter is on how you eat.

Consider raising the bar on what and how you eat. Increasing a skill level is an ongoing theme throughout this book—developing social adeptness, making humor more prevalent, and deepening your understanding and practice of mindful living. Learn how to plan and prepare delicious and healthy meals and snacks. Check out the all-new interactive meal planner and grocery list features on diabetesfoodhub.org, which make planning meals, tracking nutrition, and shopping for groceries easy.

Learn how to use spices and herbs instead of large amounts of salt and fats to make food taste good. Eat mindfully, paying attention to what you are eating and drinking, enjoying the experience, eating slowly to get the most out of each taste. (Research has shown that people who eat slowly are less likely to be obese. Those who eat quickly are twice as likely to be overweight than those who eat slowly.) As the Zen master might say, be in your mouth, where the action is. When you eat fast and do not pay attention to smell and taste, you will eat more and enjoy it less. By eating slowly and savoring every bite, you will need less food to be satisfied, and your heightened awareness will add pleasure to your meals. Also, pay attention to the size of the plates you are using. Research has shown that people who use small plates eat fewer calories.

Most of us enjoy going out to eat, which can pose challenges for people with diabetes because you have less control over how the food is prepared than in your kitchen. In Chapter 6, you learned about the need to be assertive, to speak on your own behalf, for what you want or need. When you are order-ing in a restaurant, ask how a dish is prepared. If you are not satisfied, ask if it can be done differently. Restaurants want your business, and they usually are willing to make modifications to suit their customers. For instance, a sauce or dressing can be served on the side, so you can determine how much or how little you use. Do not assume anything; ask **mindful questions** and be in control.

A primary principle for this book is that there is a belief or beliefs underlying what we do or don't do. Be mindful of the frame or frames you have for eating. Do you believe it is unfair that you can't eat that lobster thermidor without unhealthy consequences? Do you feel deprived when you pass on the cheesecake that others are having? Is your frame, "It isn't fair" or "I can't do this"? If the frame is working against you, change to one that works. Begin with these **mindful questions**:

MQ	*What are my frames for eating, and are they downers?*
	How can I reframe the problem to validate my ability and determination to eat sensibly and feel good about it?

A patient at the Johns Hopkins Comprehensive Diabetes Center shared this frame for maintaining control of what she eats: "I'm not going to put anything in my mouth that's going to take me out!" This is perhaps a bit dramatic, but it says in effect that the reason she doesn't eat certain foods is not because she can't, but rather because she chooses not to. With this frame, she does not feel deprived; to the contrary, she is proud of the strength of her willpower in taking care of herself.

EXERCISING SENSIBLY

The Centers for Disease Control and Prevention recommend leisure-time exercise at least twice weekly. The agency advises adults to engage in "moderate-intensity aerobic physical activity for at least 150 minutes per week" or "vigorous-intensity aerobic physical activity for at least 75 minutes per week," or any combination of the two. Their guidelines for children and adolescents are 60 minutes or more of physical activity daily. Most of the 60 or more minutes a day should be either moderate- or vigorous-intensity aerobic physical activity and should include vigorous-intensity physical activity at least 3 days a week.

Exercising regularly and moderately can have numerous positive benefits, such as:
- Burning calories
- Managing weight
- Increasing strength and flexibility
- Improving balance
- Strengthening and toning muscles
- Aiding treatment of osteoarthritis
- Decreasing total cholesterol and increasing HDL cholesterol (the "good" cholesterol)
- Lowering blood pressure
- Reducing risk of hypertension and arthritis
- Reducing risk of heart disease and stroke
- Reducing risk of obesity
- Reducing muscular tension
- Reducing resting heart rate over time
- Releasing stress
- Reducing blood glucose level

There are circumstances for which exercise poses a risk:
- Exercise can worsen existing problems with the eyes, kidneys, and nerves.
- High-intensity exercise can cause blood glucose to rise.
- Blood glucose can drop too low during or after exercise of long duration.
- Blood glucose can drop significantly up to 30 hours after exercise.
- For someone with type 1 diabetes, the presence of ketones in the urine or blood shows a dangerous lack

of insulin and the immediate need for more insulin. Exercise, at this time, will only burn more fat and produce more ketones, putting the person at risk for diabetic ketoacidosis (DKA), a serious medical emergency.

Given the risks, it is important to be mindful of your blood glucose level before exercising and to know how you tend to respond to exercise so you do not put yourself at risk.

Generally, exercise is an effective way to immediately lower blood glucose levels. The change varies from person to person, so you will need to check a few times before and after working out to gauge its effects on your blood glucose level. I had a young patient at the Johns Hopkins Comprehensive Diabetes Center who knew almost exactly how much he needed to exercise to lower his blood glucose level by a specific amount. It was his primary means of glucose management.

The value of exercising goes beyond the physical benefits. Working out reduces emotional tension and stress. It also improves mood and can alleviate symptoms of depression. Exercising regularly increases self-esteem. Individuals who keep fit tend to feel good about themselves.

Despite the tremendous benefits of exercising regularly, many people who want and need to work out are not able to continue an exercise program for long. The barriers to keeping a commitment to regular exercise include lack of time, fatigue, and, for many, exercise is just not fun. If any of these issues has prevented you from working out regularly, here are some ideas that might help.

Not Enough Time to Exercise

Cartoonist Randy Glasbergen created a cartoon in which a doctor who has just examined his patient says, "What fits your busy schedule better? Exercising 1 hour a day or being dead 24 hours a day?" We seem to have time for all sorts of nonsense, which is why there is no time left for doing the important things. If you believe that exercising is important to your health—important to managing your diabetes—there will be time. If you believe you do not have the time, ask these *mindful questions*:

MQ | *How much time do I spend watching television, surfing the Internet, playing computer games, or text messaging?*

Are any of these activities more important than taking good care of my health?

How can I frame this issue to motivate me to make exercise a priority in my lifestyle?

Try this frame: "There are few things I do that are more important to my well-being than to exercise regularly." Or you might use the punch line from Glasbergen's cartoon.

Not Enough Energy to Exercise

There may be times now and then when you are too tired to work out, but if fatigue is a frequent or constant problem, something is going on that needs to be addressed. If you are constantly on the go and don't balance that expenditure of energy with adequate play and rest, you won't have anything left for exercise.

It might be helpful to tell a close relative or friend that you are always tired and listen to their feedback. Sometimes others see us more clearly than we can see ourselves. A variety of medical conditions, such as a lack of essential vitamins and minerals (iron deficiency, for example), can cause fatigue. Poor blood glucose management will drain the energy right out of you. Just being out of shape can account for low energy, a problem that regular exercise can resolve. If you are tired a lot of the time, tell your doctor about it.

There's No Fun in Exercise

This is certainly a frequently expressed opinion, but exercise really can be a lot of fun. There are numerous ways to make exercise an enjoyable experience. Exercise can be a social event with friends. Join or form a regular walking group. This is a popular way to add a pleasurable dimension to your workout. Some people find that dancing to some lively music makes the physical grind more agreeable.

With current technology, there are some very creative ways to combine pleasure with a good workout. With a variety of electronic devices, you can listen to your favorite music or an audiobook while walking or using a treadmill. There are numerous apps on the Internet about exercising—apps that are designed to inform, train, motivate, and provide performance feedback to the user. In addition, there are apps specifically for seniors, women, and children.

Some Tips for Making Exercise Sensible
- Train, don't strain. Begin working out at a level that is consistent with your physical ability. If your starting point is questionable, start at a safe (low) level and gradually increase your program. If there are medical issues to consider, consult with your physician.
- Learn all you can to make exercising a healthy experience. Determine when to eat before and after working out. Learn about the upper and lower limits of your target zone for aerobic exercise. Learn how to stretch your muscles and warm up before working out and how to cool down after exercising. You may need help in planning a healthy exercise program. Information is available at public libraries, on the Internet, and at athletic clubs.
- Be aware of how your body responds to exercise. Because working out alters blood glucose levels, it is

important to know to what extent the exercise affects it. For example, someone on a regimen of premeal insulin might chose to modify a dose if intending to exercise. In fact, some insulin-sensitive individuals with type 1 diabetes may have to have a snack during prolonged or intense exercise. Understanding how your glucose level responds to physical activity will protect you from having a hypoglycemic episode due to exercising, and it can be helpful in managing your glucose level.

- Always have a fast-acting source of carbohydrate available (for example, glucose tabs) in case you develop hypoglycemia while exercising.

- Remember that exercise does not have to be harsh or vigorous to be effective. Starting at the most conservative level will be a step to better health—physically and mentally. Worldwide research published in *The Blue Zones: Lessons for Living Longer from the People Who've Lived the Longest* (4) has found that exercise is a primary factor in living a long life. But it was not vigorous exercise that made the difference. In the villages and rural areas where people lived the longest, there were no health clubs or fancy exercise equipment. The people walked or rode their bikes—and they were not in a hurry.

- Slow and steady may actually win the race. High-impact exercise, such as running marathons, gives joint cartilage a severe pounding. In the long run, low-impact exercise— walking, swimming, yoga, tai chi—may be a wiser choice. Many of the people in the "blue zones" and who tend to live the longest get their exercise by gardening.

- Set up your own tentative exercise program. Begin with what you will do at the start and how you intend to increase your activity and when. Set a goal and develop a program for reaching it (see Chapter 4: A Goal-Minded Approach to Behavior Change). You can always revise the program if it is too hard or too easy, but putting your plan on paper will help you stay on track, evaluate how you are doing, and decide what you will do next.

- If there are any questions or concerns about exercising, consult with your doctor first.

MAINTAINING A BALANCED LIFESTYLE

Living at the extremes—doing too much or not enough— is an invitation to a stressful existence. Being out of balance is stressful. Living in a state of imbalance is living in a state of instability. It drains energy and causes wear and tear on the body and mind.

Although our jobs can be very rewarding, the workplace can be a major source of stress. Today many companies are downsizing; the workers who remain are required to pick up the slack by working longer and harder. Also, dual-career couples can experience considerable pressure from their jobs and go home to find each other in similar distress.

It is essential to balance work with adequate rest and play, to reenergize with sufficient sleep and other restful behavior, such as meditation or prayer. Reading, doing crossword puzzles, painting, and going to the movies, the theater, or a concert are ways to play that conserve and restore energy. In writing this edition of my book, I took brief breaks and ended each writing session by playing a few games of scrabble on my iPad, which provided a pleasant balance to the focus and intensity of the project.

It is important, too, to be balanced internally. Thinking at the extremes (everything is either right or wrong, black or white, good or bad), personalizing (blaming yourself for everything that goes wrong), or exaggerating (making things worse than they are) can cause extreme stress. A major value of practicing *mindfulness* is to recognize these forms of imbalance and to restore balance by reframing the faulty beliefs. Letting go is a powerful way to correct a troubling imbalance in thinking and believing (see Chapter 9: The Frame of Letting Go). Letting go of a long-term grudge or grievance as opposed to holding on to the anger it provokes restores balance and relieves stress. Letting go of bad habits, behaviors, and resentments about your medical condition eliminates imbalances that otherwise generate stress and other undesirable consequences.

DEVELOPING AND USING SUPPORT

In dealing with the continual demands of diabetes, there will be times when you feel somewhat overwhelmed—times when the support of someone "special" is needed. That special person(s) may be a family member or a friend or coworker who is distinguished by his or her understanding of the basics of diabetes and the ability to calm and comfort you in the process of resolving the current crisis—without judging you. Hopefully, when you need the support, you will make contact without hesitation. Support can come from the opposite direction when this caring individual realizes that you are experiencing an extreme blood glucose level and intervenes on your behalf.

Personal and professional support are important aspects of a healthy lifestyle. The comfort and wisdom of others are invaluable resources for taking good care of yourself. Sound advice and a warm hug relieve stress, a vital component of successful self-care.

If there is a diabetes support group in your area, you would do well to attend it. Being with others who are or who have faced the same challenges can be rewarding. In Chapter 12 (Anticipate It), you are advised to have someone at work— or in your college dorm or any place where you might have an episode of hypoglycemia—who will watch for and take appropriate action in case you become disoriented by an extremely low blood glucose level.

Another useful source of support is the Internet, but it is essential that you make certain that the provider of the information is legitimate. In Chapter 14, authentic websites and other Internet resources are listed. Also, check your local hospital or health clinic for information about nearby support group activities.

Do not take on diabetes by yourself. Just as being too dependent is not healthy, being too independent is not in your best interest. Being connected to others is a basic human need. Being connected to healthy, trustworthy relatives, friends, and coworkers is a blessing.

What Can I Do to Create a Rich, Healthy, and Happy Lifestyle?

LIVE ON PURPOSE

Living purposefully—making everyday decisions and choices based on your values, needs, and interests—begins with setting meaningful goals by which to live. You will achieve what you want when you have clearly defined what your purposes are and then act consistently with the measures you have set.

To be happy and fulfilled, your life has to have meaning. For life to be meaningful, it must be consistent with the goals you have chosen for yourself. Living without purpose is living aimlessly; it is surrendering your destiny to chance. Numerous studies have shown the value of living with meaning. A 2005 study of more than 12,000 individuals found that those who believed their lives had meaning had significantly lower rates of cancer and heart disease than those who did not. In other research, people who attended a church, synagogue, or mosque at least four times a month were less likely to display risky behavior, be depressed, or experience chronic stress.

For many, retirement from work can be stressful because work had been such an important part of their lives. Another study of more than 12,000 retirees found a 51% greater risk of mortality than for those who continued to work. In another study of 3,500 people who retired at age 55, the rate of mortality was twice as high as for those who continued to work. These studies suggest that it is essential to have a reason to get up each day, and for many, that reason is to go to work. If retirement is imminent, begin planning a purposeful future absent of work. Whether it is work or some other activity, doing something that has meaning and that is purpose-driven is the foundation of a rich, healthy, and happy lifestyle.

A healthy lifestyle is guided by clearly defined purposes, each serving as your personal GPS (global positioning system) and guiding you in the pursuit of health and happiness. To assess the quality of your lifestyle, start with these *mindful questions*:

MQ	*Does my lifestyle have meaning?*
	If not, what would make my life meaningful? What is missing?
	Even if my lifestyle is meaningful, can I make it more so?

There are many ways to make life meaningful. First, taking responsibility for your health has deep meaning. It is essential for a rich and gratifying lifestyle. In addition, doing what is interesting and worthwhile adds meaning to life. Work and participating in religious activities tend to be meaningful for many individuals. For many, doing something creative—for example, painting, doodling, writing poetry, or scrapbooking—brings lifestyle to a higher level. Doing volunteer work or serving those who are less fortunate than yourself can bring the highest order of meaning to life.

With regard to taking responsibility for your health, consider these *mindful questions*:

MQ	*Is my lifestyle consistent with good diabetes care?*
	Is there anything about my lifestyle that works against good glycemic management?

*Day by day, what is my primary
purpose for living well with diabetes?*

*Will this purpose lead me to taking
the best care of myself?*

Give careful consideration to your primary purpose for
living well with diabetes. You might be tempted to conclude
that it is to avoid extreme hypoglycemia and hyperglycemia,
certainly a worthwhile purpose. But this goal will not result
in the best care possible. Consider this alternative: "All of the
things I want for myself and those I love depend on my being in
the best health possible, which means managing all aspects of
my diabetes. This is my primary purpose."

Living with purpose is not limited to life in general. It is as
important—and as rewarding—to live the everyday matters
with purpose. An appointment with a doctor is a good example.
Have you ever left a doctor's office feeling frustrated or
confused? Have you left without the answer to a question you
intended to ask but didn't because the doctor dominated the
conversation? If you had spent a brief time before the appointment defining the purpose of the meeting for you, you would
have left the doctor's office satisfied that you had gotten what
you wanted. Make your everyday choices purposeful ones.

MQ

What is my purpose for today?

What is my purpose for this moment?

*Does working too much and sleeping
too little fulfill a purpose for me?
If not, why am I doing it?*

*Does what I am doing on purpose
make me happy? If not, what do
I need to change about my purpose
to make me happy?*

But even having a clear purpose in mind, you may still find it easy to be distracted and act in a way that is inconsistent with what you intended to do. Refer to the box below for a simple but powerful model for staying on purpose and not being pulled off track.

You will get the most from life when your choices are guided by mindful, well-chosen purposes. This mindful approach to how you live your life eliminates being trapped by faulty beliefs and old patterns of behavior that are diminishing life's experiences. It gives meaning to every step you take and every choice you make. You will find helpful guidelines for setting and achieving your personal goals in Chapter 4.

BE GRATEFUL

Gratitude, a feeling of thankfulness, is one of the richest experiences you can have. The feeling of gratefulness is a wonderfully positive emotion. Research indicates that a pattern of feeling thankful has numerous lasting benefits:

- Better overall health
- Fewer physical symptoms
- More energy
- Broader social connections
- Stronger marriages
- Sounder sleep patterns
- Higher income
- Less stress

STAYING ON PURPOSE

In any situation in which you are not sure what to do, follow these steps:

1. Answer the *mindful question*: What is my purpose in this situation?

2. Answer the *mindful question*: What do I need to do right now to move toward my purpose?

3. Do it!

And the possibilities for being grateful are endless. When we exercise the ability to choose what we pay attention to, the opportunity to feel grateful is everywhere. Unfortunately, it is common to become attached to our disappointments, to what went wrong, to perceived failures, and to unfulfilled expectations. Being fixed on the hardships can blind one from reasons to be grateful.

So the task is the same as it has been for changing any situation for the better. In reframing a faulty belief— letting go of a troublesome behavior or solving a problem— the first step is to recognize that what is happening is not in your best interest. The next step is to be mindful of the choices that will enable you to change the situation for the better.

Perhaps you have been recently diagnosed with diabetes and are wondering how you could possibly feel grateful for this hardship. Maybe you are thinking about the restrictions that have been imposed on you and the complications that are associated with diabetes. To shift your attention to what you can feel grateful for, ask these *mindful questions*:

MQ | *Is it useful to focus on what makes me sad, angry, or fearful?*

Looking around, what can I see to be grateful for? (There are numerous facets of life that we take for granted: the food on the table each day, clean running water, the availability of essential medications, the freedom to worship or not, transportation, a roof overhead, electricity, music, the beauty of nature, the five senses . . . just to name a few.)

Looking inward, what can I be grateful for about me? (Consider these possibilities: A kind, charitable nature; a compassion toward others; my accomplishments; a determination to do well, to learn, and to grow; an ability to make friends.)

Thinking about my life, what can I remember to be grateful for? (Some experiences to contemplate are a joyful marriage, raising a loving family, a successful career, accomplishments in sports or other venues.)

What about diabetes can I be thankful for? (As a start, ponder a loving, supportive family; their patience and tolerance when you made a mistake; insulin, medications, and medical advancements; learning self-control; a caring, competent team of professional care providers.)

If you are able to feel grateful about your surroundings, about yourself, or about something from your past, that is wonderful. If not, make a commitment to finding ways to be grateful. See it as a choice you have at every moment and with any circumstances. To help you in this endeavor, here are a variety of ways to feel and express your gratitude:

- Mindfully develop an appreciation for small gifts in the moment. It may be a smile, a compliment—the small pleasures and blessings of every day.

- Keep a gratitude journal. On a daily basis, record what did or did not happen that you can be thankful for.
- If keeping a journal is not your style, then pause each night before you go to sleep and think of three things from the day that made you feel grateful.
- Each day, plan to do something kind for someone, even if you don't know the receiver and even if you may never be thanked for your good deed.
- Give small gifts freely. It can be a smile, compliment, hug, or kind word.
- Help someone who needs it. Maybe it is going to the grocery store for someone who is ill or volunteering at a hospital, hospice, or soup kitchen. There are few experiences that are more gratifying than serving someone less fortunate than yourself.
- Donate to worthy charities as best you can. Remember, you cannot give what you haven't received.

There is another way to feel grateful. Think about a misfortune you experienced, and find something in it to be grateful about. Your first reaction may be, "What, are you kidding?" No, it is not a joke.

On July 20, 1966, Lt. Edward L. Hubbard was flying a reconnaissance mission over Vietnam when his plane was hit by enemy fire and crashed. Hubbard parachuted to the ground and was captured. He spent over 6 years in a prison camp, often referred to as the "Hanoi Hilton," during which time he was routinely starved, tortured, and put into solitary confinement. He lived on approximately 300 calories a day, consisting of a small bowl of rice and two bowls of soup made of boiled weeds. At 5 months of captivity and on his 28th day of solitary confinement, he recalled the story of the man who felt sorry for himself because he had no shoes, until he met a man who had no feet. With this recollection, Lt. Hubbard concluded that probably more than 99% of the world was having a worse day than he was having. And from that day on, he vowed to never allow himself to have another bad day.

Now a motivational speaker, retired Colonel Hubbard attributes his reasoning on that dreadful day as a key to his survival. In the worst of situations, he was able to find something to be thankful for—something uplifting to offset his dismal circumstances.

I am reminded of a conversation with Carrie Grady, who has type 1 diabetes. She was a freshman at Johns Hopkins University when she called me because she was interested in pursuing a career as a care provider in the field of diabetes. In one of our discussions, I asked her if there was anything about having diabetes for which she could be thankful. Without hesitation, she said, "Yes. There are reasons to be grateful about having diabetes." She told me that dealing with diabetes had heightened her concerns for others. She had been self-centered before the onset of her condition, but now she was motivated by the plight of others. With her birthday approaching, her mother had asked her what she wished for. She said that it "was not so much to be cured, but to help others" who were similarly afflicted. Carrie noted, too, that having diabetes helped her overcome a fear of needles, which initially had been a very stressful matter for her.

BE CREATIVE

To create is to bring something new into being. Using your imagination to form a new idea or using your imagination and hands to produce a new object is one of the most rewarding experiences possible. To create something from your own mind and hands that did not exist before can be very gratifying. The act of creating is an effective form of self-expression. It can be a pleasant and fascinating experience. Furthermore, it is always possible.

Doodling, drawing, painting, beading, knitting, quilting, wood carving, playing a musical instrument, and writing poetry are only a few of the numerous crafts and art forms you can enjoy. A creative activity is a healthy distraction from physical and mental discomfort. It is a choice that shifts attention to something exciting, challenging, and ultimately rewarding as opposed to being stuck in a stressful mood or worse. Being creative is an excellent way to counter the weight of dealing with diabetes; creative activity helps to bring balance to lifestyle. Being creative is a safe, adaptive way to escape from life's dissatisfactions.

I enjoy creating haiku, an unrhymed verse form of Japanese origin having three lines containing five, seven, and five syllables, respectively. Here is one of my favorites:

> *Instant vacation*
> *It's right there under your nose*
> *A big belly laugh*

If you are thinking that being creative is not a choice for you because you do not have any creative ability, it may be that you have chosen not to have it. Anyone can be creative. Being creative does not depend on skills and intelligence, although those traits will affect how creativity is expressed. Some common barriers to being creative are 1) unrealistic expectations, 2) impatience, 3) being overly competitive, 4) having an irrational need to please others, and 5) a faulty belief, such as, "I don't have artistic ability."

Learning to be creative starts with the right frames: "I can do it. It does not have to be profound or perfect. It just has to be fun." From this optimistic perspective, it takes only commitment and practice to achieve your goal. Remember that whenever you are in the pursuit of an objective, it is important to be realistic. The greatest artists in history did not start out producing masterpieces; they struggled repeatedly to improve their art form.

Pick a craft that is appealing, and do some research on how to get started. Your local library will have a selection of books on any art form you choose. Not surprisingly, the Internet can also provide a broad spectrum of information about any craft. The Internet is also a source for making contact with others who practice the skill of your choice. Stores that sell craft supplies offer training in a variety of hobbies. Stores that sell art supplies and specialty enterprises, such as wool shops, can be excellent resources. Be patient and leave your ego somewhere else. Certainly, you can expect to make progress, but your assessments need to be realistic and reasonable.

BE SPIRITUAL

Spirituality is usually associated exclusively with religion, but there is another level to spirituality that is important to a healthy lifestyle. For many people, a religion-based spirituality gives their lives a deep sense of meaning. However, there are many people for whom religion does not work or is not appealing. In *The Art of Happiness: A Handbook for Living* (5), the inimitable spiritual leader of Tibet, His Holiness the Dalai Lama, coined the term for a second level of spirituality: "basic spirituality." He described it as living the basic human qualities of goodness, kindness, compassion, and caring. Basic spirituality is the practice of inner discipline rooted in a calm and stable state of mind. It is a level of mindfulness that raises us above ourselves and connects us to something larger—to other people, to the environment, and to responsibility for the future. It is turning away from materialism and consumerism and reaching for the highest values.

The values of basic spirituality are numerous. Practicing the principles of this level of spirituality is exercising control over negative emotions and patterns of behavior that do not work well. As you develop and strengthen the qualities of kindness and caring, you are able to resist the temptation to act in a mean-spirited manner, with all of its unpleasant consequences. When your mind is calm and stable, you are not going to lose control and act in a destructive way. Drawing on your spirituality is rising above frustrations and resentments; it is a powerful way to prevent the onset of stress that is caused by inappropriate reactions to the behavior of others.

Every situation—from the mundane to the profound— is an opportunity to practice basic spirituality. Looking at a photograph of a deceased loved one and having a warm, loving feeling is practice. Walking in a park, in the woods, or on a beach and simply celebrating the natural wonder of what you see is practicing spirituality. Being kind to someone who has not been kind to you is practicing basic spirituality.

Finding an inspiring meaning for a personal crisis may not be easy, but can anything be more rewarding? It is the mindset for seeking the comfort and rewards of spirituality and finding deeper meaning in the face of life's challenges.

How Can I Assess My Lifestyle Choices?

A mindful approach to any issue begins with one or more *mindful questions*. Whether it is making a change, solving a problem, assessing a situation, or evaluating oneself, asking the right questions stimulates the reflection necessary for well-informed decisions. Here are some *mindful questions* to consider in your pursuit of a healthy and happy lifestyle:

MQ
> *Does my lifestyle help me manage my diabetes?*
>
> *Is my lifestyle meaningful?*
>
> *Is my lifestyle purposeful?*
> *Is my lifestyle balanced?*
>
> *Does my lifestyle make me happy?*
>
> *Is being grateful a purpose in my life?*
>
> *What can I add to my life that I would be grateful for?*
>
> *Does doing something creative enrich my life?*

> *What can I do today to be kinder than I was yesterday?*
>
> *Is my lifestyle as "low stress" as possible?*
>
> *Is my lifestyle causing me or someone else harm?*
>
> *What might happen if I made a commitment to practice "basic spirituality" for 1 month?*

As you reflect on each of these questions, you will learn which aspects of your lifestyle need further consideration and change. Each "no" leads to other *mindful questions*:

MQ
> *Why not?*
>
> *What do I have to do to make the answer "yes"?*

If this line of reflection does not work, try the problem-solving techniques described in Chapter 11 for each part of your lifestyle that is not at its best.

For example, if your answer to the first *mindful question*—Does my lifestyle help me manage my diabetes?—was "no," the next step is to identify what about the way you are living is working against managing diabetes. Think about what you need to change to get your lifestyle in line with good diabetes management. Reflect on the answers to these *mindful questions*:

MQ
> *Which aspects of my lifestyle are not helping me to manage my diabetes?*

> *For each negative aspect, what is the problem or problems to be solved to get my lifestyle in order?*

What do the answers to these questions indicate about changing the way you are living your life for the purpose of achieving better diabetes management? If your lifestyle is out of balance—if, for example, you are too busy and make little time for rest and play—what changes are needed to meet your end point? Follow the model for problem solving (see Chapter 11). With relentless determination, consider each issue and every possibility for change. Jot down your thoughts, and ultimately draw a map, beginning with where you are and ending with where you need to be. Between the beginning and end points, list everything you have to do to get there. See Chapter 4 (A Goal-Minded Approach to Behavior Change) for help in drawing the map and ensuring that you will succeed in making each change you recognize in this process.

What Are the Barriers to a Healthy Lifestyle?

There are three primary barriers to living well: 1) not knowing any better, 2) mindlessly repeating learned patterns of behavior that do not work, and 3) mindlessly acting on faulty beliefs. A disordered lifestyle produces one stress after another. By the time you have finished reading this book, you will be well on your way to thinking, feeling, and acting mindfully. It won't always be easy, but it will always be possible.

Keep in mind that it is never too late to benefit from a healthy lifestyle. A study reported in *Science* (July 2007) has determined that there are benefits from making the way you live healthier, even later in life. Take charge and make it happen—the payoff will be huge no matter how old you are when you change your lifestyle for the better. The healthier your lifestyle, the less stress there will be; the less stress, the better your diabetes management.

PART 3

Key Tools for Mastering Stress

CHAPTER 8

Reframing

Everyone is a product of their personal beliefs. Unfortunately, many are also victims of their beliefs. What you do or don't do is determined by what you believe. You select a particular restaurant or movie because you believe it will be pleasurable. You choose not to ride the roller coaster because you believe it is dangerous. You draw blood from your finger several times a day because you believe that not doing it can put you in harm's way.

You may think of your beliefs as an attitude ("I just don't like Greek food") or value ("I keep all of my money in the bank; no stocks or bonds for me"). However, upon close examination, you will realize that each of these positions developed from experiences or messages from the past that became beliefs about what to expect if you do this or that. A bad experience at a Greek restaurant may become a belief that Greek restaurants are to be avoided. A relative who lived through the Great Depression and spoke of experiencing great financial loss in the stock market may pass on a negative belief about investments. Think about it. Why are you reading this book? Is it because you believe that reducing your stress will help you better manage your diabetes and you expect that reading it will help you achieve both objectives?

Beliefs are generalizations—interpretations of life's experiences that become attitudes, points of view, expectations, and values. Beliefs are the perceived truths by which you live. Your beliefs become the basis of your reality. They determine how you think, feel, and behave. They determine the quality of your life. Consider this parable about the difference between heaven and hell:

> *It has been said that those who go to heaven spend all of eternity studying the holy books. Those in hell spend eternity studying the holy books.*

We have all experienced situations that have been heaven for some and hell for others. The difference is determined by differences in perceptions and differences based on individual beliefs. What you perceive about the world around you is an interaction of immediate data from the senses and other information accumulated and stored in the brain from previous experiences. These interactions can be very complicated and twisted, becoming misleading, troublesome beliefs. When reactions to beliefs are automatic, mindless activity, you risk becoming the victim of ill-informed convictions and you surrender the power of making informed choices. You become a passenger—rather than the driver—in your life. With purposeful willpower and commitment, you can make certain that your experiences are driven by sound, informed beliefs. With an alert and reflective approach to life, you claim the power that eliminates the risks of mindless, irrational perceptions of your experiences.

Reframing is changing what you believe about something and, thereby, claiming control of this powerful force in your life. It is being mindful about the beliefs that are driving your thoughts, feelings, and behavior and choosing to change a belief when it does not work for you. Nothing is likely to cause you more stress than acting mindlessly on your beliefs. Nothing is more likely to reduce your level of stress than to reframe faulty beliefs.

Living mindfully is the fundamental principle that underlies each of the techniques and tools described in this book. Practitioners of mindfulness are fully present in the moment, aware of what is happening internally and externally, neither overly reactive nor overwhelmed by what is happening and their perceptions are without judgment. To practice mindful living is to practice creating space for oneself—space to think, space to breathe, space between ourselves and our reactions. That space can make a critical difference between winning and losing. Viktor Frankl (6), a renowned author who survived the Holocaust, wrote that, "Between stimulus and response, there is a space. In that space is our power to choose our response. In our response lies our growth and our freedom."

A frame is a belief. I use the word "frame" for "belief" because using the image of taking down a frame and hanging a new one in its place—the act of reframing—gives the action a visual boost. When you challenge a belief, you can envision taking one frame down and hanging another frame in its place. The image adds a visual dimension to the process, making it more mindful. Being mindful opens the door to recognizing a faulty belief and reframing it with a rational one.

How Did I Get My Beliefs?

From our earliest experiences—even before we have developed a language for representing what happened—we begin to acquire beliefs about ourselves and the world around us. Given their limited capacities, children are basically receptors of information and values. The very young have little, if any, ability to assess or challenge the worth of what they see and hear. Consequently, a child's beliefs depend largely on the wisdom and health of those who feed their viewpoints to the youngster. Beliefs are formed directly and indirectly.

A child who makes an innocent mistake and is called "stupid" may develop the belief that he or she is a stupid person, especially when the putdowns are frequent. When the parents of a child diagnosed with diabetes convey a sense of guilt or shame, the child may believe that he or she is defective or inadequate. If a parent is anxious or angry about the diabetes, the child may conclude that he or she has done something wrong and is to blame for the parent's distress. The child who is ignored by significant others will believe that he or she is unworthy of the attention and affection of others. The child of parents who separate is at risk of believing that it was his or her fault—that if he or she had been a better son or daughter, the separation would not have happened.

The process of acquiring a belief can be even more complex. Jane was 8 years old when she was diagnosed with diabetes. Although her parents were very supportive and positive about the situation, Jane knew that her grandfather had a leg amputated because of his diabetes. She had witnessed dramatic incidents when paramedics were summoned because he had lost consciousness because of extremely low blood glucose levels. Although her parents assured Jane that she would be alright, she could not stop the memories of her grandfather's ordeal. Consequently, Jane believed that she was doomed to the same fate.

In the classes at the Johns Hopkins Comprehensive and Suburban Hospital Diabetes Centers, I tell this story:

At the age of 9 or 10, I was with my father at a public bath facility. We were in shower stalls next to one another. I was washing and innocently whistling, and my father hollered at me. It was clear that he was annoyed by the sound of my whistling, and his disapproval was unnerving. Many years later, I am still self-conscious about whistling in the presence of anyone. The frame that formed from that experience was, "It is annoying and dangerous for me to whistle." If I started to whistle, I immediately looked around to see if anyone was in hearing range. But when I learned the power of reframing, I was able to recognize the irrationality of the belief and reframe it with, "Just whistle; my whistling is not bad! If anyone doesn't like it, so what?"

What is so fascinating about this experience is that although it was such a small trauma, it created a negative belief that persisted for a very long time. Being self-conscious persisted until I was able to mindfully change the frame and whistle to my satisfaction.

The behavior of parents is not the only source of our beliefs. A relative or neighbor—and especially our childhood peers— can convey a message that is perceived to be true when it is not so. The youngster with type 1 diabetes, who goes to the school nurse to inject insulin, can be the target of teasing and demeaning comments by an uninformed or discontent peer. Nonetheless, the unkind remarks can become a faulty belief that fuels self-debasing feelings for the individual who was unjustly criticized.

How Can My Beliefs Affect Me?

What you believe determines how you think, feel, and act in response to what is happening at any given time. Think about it. Is there anything you do or don't do that is not rooted in a belief or beliefs about the matter at hand? Attitudes, view- points, values, and expectations are all based on what you believe. If someone invited you to go to see a western movie, you might say, "No thank you. I really don't like cowboy movies." Without diminishing the truth of that response, you might also have said that you don't believe that you would enjoy going to a western film. Or perhaps you believe that going to a cowboy movie is just not "cool."

You surely are familiar with the cliché "seeing is believing." Well, how about the opposite, "believing is seeing"? Or, as a participant in one of the diabetes center classes put it, "You'll see it when you believe it."

All of our perceptions begin with the senses and end with an individual impression or understanding that is determined after filtering through our personal belief system. From a purely sensory perspective, the cowboy movie is likely to be the same for all: everyone sees the hero chasing the bad guy on horseback. Perceptions of the action might be very different, or even contrary. One observer might be elated that the Indian who is being chased will be captured or killed. After all, he had brought harm to the settlers. Another observer, however, might view the scene with sadness as she thinks about the injustices that had been brought upon the American Indian as settlers took claim of their territories. She believes that the settlers deserve their fate and hopes that the fleeing Indian will escape.

The placebo effect is a dramatic example of the power of our beliefs. A placebo is a substance, device, or procedure that has a beneficial effect that cannot be accounted for by any direct physical action. The term "placebo" comes from the Latin, meaning, "I shall please." In a multitude of studies, individuals have been given an inactive substance, such as a sugar pill, and were told it was a medication developed for the relief of a particular medical problem. These studies often resulted in significant relief from a variety of symptoms, including depression, anxiety, pain, nausea, and vomiting. Research has also shown that a placebo might produce temporary relief from illnesses such as arthritis, hypertension, headache, peptic ulcer, and hay fever. Here is an interesting example of the placebo effect:

Research was conducted to test the value of constricting an artery in the thorax to relieve angina. One group of patients had the procedure done, while a second group was anesthetized but only had their skin cut very slightly. The second group did not have an artery constricted. Both groups were told that constricting the artery would relieve the chest pain they were having as a result of chronic heart ischemia. A total of 80% of the group who did not have the procedure experienced relief; only 40% of the group who had the procedure had a beneficial outcome.

The "nocebo" effect is the opposite and is very important in terms of stress management. The term is derived from the Latin, meaning "I will harm." In this case, there is a harmful result that cannot be explained by a direct physical intervention.

In a study of what women believed about their health with regard to their heart, those women who believed they were prone to heart disease were nearly four times as likely to die from heart disease as women with similar risk factors— high blood pressure, obesity, and/or high cholesterol—but who did not believe they were susceptible to coronary illness.

In another study, volunteers were told that a mild electrical current would pass through their heads. Afterwards, two-thirds of the subjects complained that they had headaches, although no electrical current was used.

In various studies, an inactive substance has had a placebo effect, relieving a wide range of symptoms. Similarly, inactive matter had the nocebo effect for many of the same symptoms. The difference was what the person was made to believe would happen upon taking the so-called medication or treatment.

The placebo and nocebo effects are noteworthy examples of how expectations affect reality. These effects add to our understanding of how beliefs can affect the quality of life. Learning about them here may bring to mind the concept of the "self-fulfilling prophecy." The idea is that if you make a prediction about the future, then it will likely happen. Of course, the link between the prediction and the outcome is the belief that it will indeed happen, and believing it, you will do everything possible to make it happen—consciously or subconsciously.

Beliefs can make you happy and strong. They can also make you sick. They are your primary source of stress. The **mindful questions** are:

MQ | *Is the belief (frame) affecting me now realistic?*

How factual is this belief? Is the evidence indisputable?

What is a fitting, constructive frame for this situation?

How Does Reframing Reduce Stress?

The focus is on beliefs that are problematic or beliefs that generate undue stress. If a belief works for you, leave it alone. However, if a belief is nonsensical or simply baseless, then you need to reframe it rationally. Beliefs can be faulty because they are based on misinformation or misunderstanding. For example, there was the man with diabetes who was having difficulty managing his blood glucose levels and finally concluded that it was his beer drinking that was the problem. He replaced the beer with fruit juices, believing that the change would help him better manage the diabetes. Obviously, because of the sugar content in fruit juices, his glucose levels did not improve; in fact, they worsened. As he suffered from more incidents of hyperglycemia, his stress and frustration grew from not understanding why what he was doing was not working.

There are beliefs that can be more troublesome. Unfortunately, beliefs are often mindlessly accepted as true even though they have no basis in fact. There are people, for example, who believe that having diabetes is shameful; they believe that they are defective. This frame for having diabetes is extremely stressful and dangerous. It sets up the self-fulfilling prophecy of self-loathing and ultimate defeat.

Operating on misbeliefs or malbeliefs—a term I coined for frames that are not only untrue but harmful—will result in serious stress, frustration, and ineffective coping with diabetes and life. But when you reframe, when you change the belief, you change what it means and what it does. At the very least, reframing neutralizes a stressful frame. At best, the new frame transforms a potentially stressful situation into a positive experience. Most important, by eliminating the stressor, the new frame gives you a new level of power over your diabetes.

Are There Other Ways that Frames Can Affect Diabetes Management?

Although many individuals with type 2 diabetes will almost surely need insulin to manage their diabetes at some point, resistance to taking insulin is common. Furthermore, although there is evidence that insulin can be more effective than oral medications for patients newly diagnosed with type 2 diabetes (patients who begin using the drug right after diagnosis), many doctors choose to avoid prescribing insulin until there is no other choice. An extensive international study investigated why people with type 2 diabetes resist taking insulin and why physicians resist prescribing insulin until absolutely necessary. The study indicated that for the patients, the barriers were pessimistic, shameful, or fear-ridden frames. Many patients believed that taking insulin was a sign that their diabetes was getting worse and that it meant they had failed in managing the disease. A negative viewpoint also held back the doctors, who believed that insulin should be avoided for as long as possible. More than half of the healthcare providers did not believe that insulin would be helpful for type 2 diabetes. These are striking examples of how faulty beliefs can impair diabetes management. It takes little thought to predict the enormous reduction in personal suffering and in health costs if type 2 diabetes patients and physicians dealt with the insulin issue on the basis of the facts.

> *Phillip has diabetes and had this frame for eating: "I cannot eat many, if not most, of the things I like so much." This frame caused Phillip a lot of stress. He was angry and pessimistic about his ability to deal with diabetes. Furthermore, when he ate what he thought was prohibited, he felt guilty and got even more agitated. But when he reframed the issue with, "I can eat anything from time to time with moderation," Phillip changed his point of view and his mood. From this new perspective, he felt confident and content that he could maintain a reasonably healthy diet most of the time.*

Don't forget: when you change the frame, you change what something means and you change what it does to you. Reframing is taking control of what you think, feel, and do. The more you are in control of what happens to you, the less stress you will experience. But when you live on automatic pilot, not paying attention to underlying, faulty beliefs, you give up control, which is an invitation for stress.

How Will I Know When to Reframe?

WHAT DO YOU BELIEVE?

Reframing is an essential skill for managing stress, and the more you know about your belief system, the better. Take time to do the exercise in the box What Are My Core Beliefs? on page 172. The exercise is designed to raise your awareness of the beliefs by which you live and, thus, give you control over them. Remember, the objective is to manage your diabetes mindfully, which means knowing what you are doing and why you are doing it. The more familiar you are with your beliefs, the sooner you will recognize when a belief needs to be reframed.

HOW WILL MY FEELINGS HELP ME REFRAME?

As pointed out before, if you touch a very hot surface, pain is the signal to move your hand away as quickly as possible to avoid further harm. As much as it might have hurt, the pain has saved you from further harm. Similarly, disturbing emotions can be a signal to be mindful and to reframe. If you feel sad, angry, or scared, use the discomfort to check the frame or frames that are driving the unpleasant feeling. The *mindful questions* are:

MQ | *What frame is causing this feeling? Is it valid?*

If the frame is invalid, what is a sound alternative?

> *If the belief is not faulty and*
> *the feeling is valid, can I still*
> *reframe the situation to*
> *improve my position?*

Reframing is not limited to replacing a faulty belief. An aspect of living mindfully is to not take anything for granted. Acting on a belief may become habitual just because it does not cause a problem, which doesn't mean there isn't a better frame to act on. Living mindfully is not only about minimizing stress; it is also about maximizing your potential and maintaining peace of mind.

WHAT IF I CANNOT LET GO OF A NEGATIVE FRAME?

Some frames stick like glue. We become attached to beliefs for many reasons. They may become deeply embedded in our minds early in life, a time when we are less discriminating or are preoccupied with other challenges in growing up. Sometimes a belief seems to be working, so it is repeated over and over again. However, what may be working in the short run may be a disaster in the bigger picture. Another trap is a frame that is working but at a very high cost. If you feel stressed and your frame is, "If I eat, I will feel better," then eating may soothe your feelings in the moment. However, in the long run, the cost of eating to soothe your feelings will cause more stress than it relieves. The *mindful questions* are:

MQ | *What is the origin of this frame?*

What evidence is there to support the validity of this frame?

The frame may be working, but at what cost?

Is there a frame that will work with less or no cost?

WHAT ARE MY CORE BELIEFS?

Your core beliefs determine what you value, fear, desire, and need. Take your time and thoughtfully write down the answers to each question.

1. What do I believe about myself in my most important relationships (with spouse, parent, sibling, lover, friend, healthcare provider)?

2. What do I believe about myself in my work?

3. What do I believe about having diabetes?

4. What do I believe when I am managing my diabetes well?

5. What do I believe when my diabetes management is not good?

6. What do I believe about my life in general (in control or not, happy or not, doing my best or not)?

7. What do I believe when something does not go well for me?

8. What do I believe when something good happens?

9. What do I believe about my future?

Looking at the answers to these questions, underscore the beliefs that do not work—the ones that are causing you stress. Each underscored belief needs to be replaced (reframed) at every opportunity because it is misdirecting your thoughts, feelings, and actions. Start now to practice reframing. Take charge.

MQ | *What is keeping me from letting go of a frame that is undesirable?*

What Can I Do to Be More Effective at Reframing?

Having raised your awareness of both your belief system and how you can use your feelings to trigger reframing an undesirable belief, you have almost everything you need to master this powerful skill. The next step is to make a commitment to reframing, so the beliefs by which you live are conscious choices.

With reframing as an ongoing purpose, the *mindful questions* are:

> MQ | *Am I in a good place now?*
>
> *If not, what is the frame that needs to be replaced?*
>
> *What frame or frames can I use here that will make this a positive experience for me?*

Keeping in mind the power of choices, the *mindful question*, when time permits, might be:

> MQ | *How many ways can I reframe the situation to make this a positive experience for me?*

(and then)

> *Which of these choices is the best right now?*

> *Andy's wife has diabetes and she is not doing well in managing the disease. Her blood glucose levels tend to run in the range of 250–350 mg/dL, and she suffers from several unpleasant symptoms, including irritability and fatigue. Frustrated and frightened, Andy often reacts angrily, accusing her of being lazy and irresponsible. His wife, in turn, withdraws emotionally and eats to comfort herself.*

In doing the core beliefs exercise, Andy became aware of beliefs he held that had been consistently limiting and stressful. He had always been intolerant of what he labeled "incompetence," an attitude that was linked to his belief that the troubles of others were a lack of willpower. The frame he imposed on his wife was, "You should be able to manage your diabetes." Another negative belief was that he was a victim of his wife's suffering. The accompanying frame was, "You are the cause of *my* misery." Committed to becoming skilled at reframing, Andy challenged the merits of the frames he had identified and gave thought to what frame or frames he could use that would be more rewarding for himself and his wife. With some reflection, he concluded that the reframes should be, "There is more to the problem than a lack of willpower. While I want her to better manager her diabetes, it is unfair to think she should be in control. Perhaps, if I cool my feelings and offer to help her to make some positive changes, it might make a difference. Lastly, I have to take responsibility for my comfort level, which will surely have a positive effect on my wife's attitude about the diabetes."

> *Allen lost his job when his employer downsized the company to decrease expenses. Shortly after, he was diagnosed with diabetes. He was furious and despondent. The combination of events triggered a set of old and intensely negative frames: "I am being punished." "I was never enough, and now, with diabetes, no one will want to hire me." "We're not going to make it." Locked into these self-defeating frames, Allen was miserable and made his wife and three children unhappy, too. He didn't know about the power of reframing. Fortunately, his wife had persuaded him to see a counselor who did know the value of challenging old, self-defeating beliefs.*

With professional help, Allen was able to make the connection between his beliefs and his troubled mental state. The next step was to challenge the soundness of each frame. He realized that the idea that he was being punished was a message he heard often as a child, when his parents attributed any misfortune to a mystical force. Also, he became aware that the belief that he was never enough became real to him after a series of rejections he experienced in his youth. He recognized, too, that there might be employers who would shun him because of the diabetes, but he was highly qualified in his field and, with a positive attitude, he could overcome the issue. When he became aware of how often and forcefully he was telling himself that he wouldn't make it, he could only laugh at himself.

Now, mindful of the problem, Allen was able to reframe his reaction to the loss of his job and the diagnosis of diabetes. The new frames were, "I'm not perfect, but I'm not so bad that I am bringing misfortune upon myself and my family. My self-worth has nothing to do with losing my job." "If someone does not hire me because I have diabetes, it will be their loss." "A lot of people in worse situations have made it, and I will, too."

Beliefs are the connecting links between an event and its outcome. There is a tendency to view experiences as a simple flow from A ⟶ B. "When we go out to eat and you order dessert (A), I get upset (B)." This scenario should be seen as having three components: A ⟶ B ⟶ C. Observing the person with diabetes ordering dessert (A) appears to trigger a distressing reaction (C), but the real culprit is the belief that, "Because you have diabetes, you should not have dessert with dinner" (B). In general, this model is as follows:

A (stimulus) ⟶ B (belief) ⟶ C (reaction) ⟶ D (dispute B)

To complete the model for taking control of your belief system, we have added another component (D): disputing and replacing a limiting or troubling belief. Keep this process in mind and practice it regularly. When your reaction to a stimulus (A) is uncomfortable (C), identify the belief (B) that is fueling your behavior (C), and challenge the validity of the belief (D). The final step is to reframe the troublesome belief with one that will change your reaction (C) to a positive one.

Let's look again at the example in which Andy is having difficulty dealing with his wife's poor glycemic management.

For Andy, the stimulus (A) was his wife's poor management and his reaction (C) was to accuse her of being irresponsible. When he disputed (D) the belief that she was acting irresponsibly (B), he became aware that his conviction was not true. He realized that her problem with control was more complex than a lack of willpower, and he was able to change his belief (B), which changed a negative situation to a positive one.

How you frame experiences affects how you think and feel about yourself and the world around you. How you frame events invites or prevents unnecessary stress. Mindfully distinguishing between good and bad frames and changing the latter is a sure prescription for success in every endeavor, including management of your diabetes.

Chapter 9 explores one of the most powerful frames for replacing self-defeating beliefs: the frame of letting go. Chapter 10 focuses on a range of positive frames as well as a variety of stress-building beliefs to avoid.

CHAPTER 9

The Frame of Letting Go

lcoholics Anonymous and other similar recovery programs define insanity as doing the same thing over and over for 20 years and expecting something different to happen. If the same bad things happen every time you open the same door, when do you wake up and try another door? When do you let go of what doesn't work and consider the possibility that something else can work?

What Is Letting Go?

Letting go is about changing the status quo for the better. It is about freeing oneself of useless or, worse, self-defeating baggage. The baggage may be a belief, an emotion, a behavior, a grudge or grievance, an interpretation of the past, or a compulsion. It is anything that you experience that is a problem for you.

The frame of letting go is a powerful stress-buster. The ability to let go is associated with several other frames:

- I am strong and wise enough to let go of what I need to let go of for my well-being.
- The choice of letting go or holding on is mine alone.
- I can tolerate the short-term discomfort and uncertainty of letting go in exchange for the long-term rewards.
- I can and will let go of any toxic clutter: the beliefs and behaviors that cause me undue hardship and pain.

Letting go is knowing that any belief or belief-driven activity can be released or changed, resulting in a different viewpoint and a different outcome. It does not mean that you extinguish or erase something; it means detaching yourself from any value or meaning it had for you. It is about letting something be what it is without giving it attention, without investing any energy in it. In most cases, the act of letting go begins with a troublesome belief.

> *Amanda was diagnosed with diabetes when she was 7 years old. She is 19 now. Her A1C is consistently in the range of 10–11%, which means that her blood glucose levels are usually very high. These levels are not a mystery, since Amanda does very little to maintain good glycemic management. She eats whatever and whenever she chooses, and her use of insulin is erratic.*

This maladaptive pattern is belief-driven—a combination of self-defeating frames: "I am damaged goods," "I hate having to take insulin," and "Even if I tried harder, it wouldn't matter in the long run." Reframing (replacing these negative frames with positive ones) starts with the belief that old, troubling frames can be replaced and that any situation can be changed by changing the frame.

When Amanda is able to let go of her pessimistic view of life with diabetes, she can reframe her condition: "I am a worthy young woman who happens to have diabetes," "Insulin is a valuable resource for controlling my blood glucose levels and reducing the risk of complications," and "The fact is that if I take better care of myself, it will make a big difference in the short and long run." With the combination of letting go of the old and choosing a new mindset, her self-defeating attitudes and behaviors will reverse, and she will be able to achieve good control. The switching of frames may be very difficult, but it is always possible.

Some remarkable examples of the power of letting go are the experiences of individuals who have survived severe hardships by resisting the temptation to accept a frame of total despair and defeat. In *Man's Search for Meaning* (6),

Viktor Frankl wrote of his experiences in a Nazi concentration camp:

> *Everything can be taken from a man but one thing, the last of the human freedoms—to choose one's attitude in any set of circumstances, to choose one's own way.*

How much did Dr. Frankl have to let go of to be open to a hopeful viewpoint while enduring the extreme deprivations and hardships of a concentration camp? Certainly, he had to let go of some conventional expectations and assumptions that could be relied on before the rise of Nazism. Anything that once had a reasonable degree of certainty before had none in the Nazi camp; nothing was certain from moment to moment. Fundamental virtues, such as fairness and justice, had to be generally abandoned. Moving from one mental zone to another requires letting go of a lot, if not all, of the connections with the zone being given up.

Arnold Beisser's story also reflects the power of letting go. At the age of 23, Arnold Beisser had graduated medical school. At age 24, he had won a national tennis championship. At 25, he contracted polio and was confined to an iron lung (a mechanical respirator that enables a person to breathe on his own) completely immobile for several months. The illness left him paraplegic and restricted to a wheelchair. In his book, *Flying Without Wings* (7), Dr. Beisser wrote, "I treated my illness as though there must be some way out of this mess." He goes on to note that he had to give up any delusion of power and "surrender gracefully" to reality. He has had a remarkable life of personal and professional achievements.

Perhaps you have heard a performance by Itzhak Perlman, an acclaimed virtuoso of the violin. Mr. Perlman has won numerous Grammy and Emmy awards, and he has performed with every major orchestra in the world. In addition, he has conducted many of the world's major orchestras. Mr. Perlman's accomplishments illustrate the effect of letting go of the impossible and investing in what can be done.

At the age of 4, Itzhak Perlman contracted polio, and, as a result, his legs are permanently paralyzed. Suffering this horrific affliction at such a young age did not deter him from pursuing the study of the violin. He has been quoted as saying, "I realized as a young boy, I did not need my legs to play the violin." At this very early age, he was able to let go of a range of functional losses and, thus, focus fully on what he was able to do. What if he believed that he had to play sandlot baseball to feel OK and could not let go of that conviction? Letting go of what is not possible opens the way to what is possible.

Everyone has "baggage": messages that we were given growing up that are misleading and perhaps irrational; patterns of behavior that are counterproductive; and programs that fire in the brain and compel actions that are useless, if not harmful. Every change for the better begins with letting go of old baggage. Put another way, you cannot learn something new without unlearning what is already in place. Albert Einstein recognized this challenge in his own life, stating, "I must be willing to give up what I am in order to become what I will be."

If expressing anger inappropriately is a problem, you need to let go of that behavior and practice a more productive way of expressing discontent. If bingeing is your reaction to frustration, you need to replace this pattern with a healthier choice. The process of unlearning and relearning begins with letting go of the faulty frames that are driving the negative actions.

Choice is power. When an unhealthy frame or behavior is held onto relentlessly, the holder is stuck in the quicksand without a choice. Choices become evident when you ask *mindful questions*:

MQ | *Which thoughts—and consequent actions— are causing me trouble?*

What is keeping me from letting go of them?

*What do I need to let go
of now to get where
I want to be?*

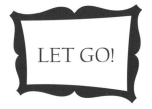

Is Letting Go Different from Giving Up?

Sometimes yes; other times no. You may have been told emphatically to *"never give up."* Perhaps you are familiar with the saying, "Quitters never win; winners never quit." But the belief "if you keep trying, you will succeed" fails when reason proves your effort is fruitless or perhaps harmful. Consider the person who has tried several times to skateboard over an object only to break a bone or two each time. Call it "letting go" or "giving up," but just stop it.

Life can be difficult. When a challenge is faced head on, you become stronger and more confident. Struggling to control diabetes requires letting go of some faulty beliefs ("I can't do it." "I'm doomed.") but not giving up.

Letting go is the process of eliminating obstacles so that you are able to meet the challenges that life presents—letting go frees you of the baggage that is holding you down. Giving up is accepting one's limitations.

How Does Letting Go Help Control Stress?

Letting go of a bad belief by reframing it is one of the most powerful stress-busters possible. Remember that stress is a reaction to a perceived threat. The way a stimulus is interpreted initiates a response. Being diagnosed with diabetes is likely to cause an emotional reaction—most commonly sadness and fear. If the diagnosis is perceived as a grave danger, the reaction will be fearful. By contrast, some individuals have reacted to the diagnosis with strong relief. Someone recently told me that she was glad it was "only diabetes" because she had felt so ill that she was certain she had cancer. However, telling someone with the ailment that it "could be worse" won't be comforting if she believes that it is the worst. Although the list of stress-producing beliefs may be endless, there are some that are very common.

LET GO OF THESE COMMON, SELF-DEFEATING BELIEFS

- Taking care of myself is being selfish.
- My first responsibility is to make the other person happy.
- Every problem is catastrophic.
- Everything that doesn't go right is my fault.
- An assumption is a fact.
- I have to have it even though I don't need it.
- All expectations are realistic.
- I have to stay in a relationship, even if it is toxic.
- A behavior is working for me regardless of the cost of my conduct.
- There is no other choice.
- It could not be any worse.
- If I ignore it, it will go away.
- It's all or nothing.
- I am the victim of someone else.
- If I give up trying (letting go of this stressful endeavor), I will be a loser.

A SPECIAL CHALLENGE FOR MANY: LETTING GO OF THE PAST

It may be true that everyone is haunted to some extent by their past. For many, the impact of the past may be relatively small or insignificant. For some, past experiences are a persistent source of stress. In more than 35 years as a psychotherapist in private practice, I have heard this belief most often: "I was never enough, and I am still not enough." This belief usually originates from experiences in which a child thinks and feels as if he or she has disappointed a parent or another significant person. Children can be very sensitive to what is happening, but they have limited ability to interpret the meaning of what is going on correctly. For example, a child who is trying to adapt to diabetes may sense a parent's anxiety about the situation but conclude that the concern about a very high blood glucose level is their disappointment with him or her. If the parents of children with diabetes separate, then those children might conclude that it is their fault because they are not "normal" and that somehow their condition caused the split-up.

These types of experiences become hardwired in the brain in the form of negative and often debilitating frames: "I'm never enough, so why try?" or "I'm never enough, but maybe I can avoid the painful criticism and rejection by doing everything possible to please everyone." The consequences of giving up or being compelled to take care of everyone but yourself will make dealing with diabetes and life in general immensely stressful. While everyone has shortcomings, the idea of not being enough is likely to be an exaggerated and distorted perception that needs to be dropped.

Another dynamic that continually creates stress is holding on to grudges and grievances from the past. Being angry with someone who hurt you is a normal, automatic reaction; holding the hurt with a vengeance is a common, self-inflicted burden. Letting go or holding on to anguish is a choice.

The challenge is to forgive the one who hurt you, which tends to be very difficult for many individuals. When faced with the idea of forgiving someone who caused considerable suffering, the reaction is likely to be, "Why should I?" The operating frame may be that the offender was the bad one and should apologize or suffer some form of punishment. The problem is that the wrongdoer has probably forgotten the event a long time ago or has written it off as insignificant; so you are the only one who is emotionally involved in this matter. Letting go of the grudge, forgiving the other, is not about letting him off the hook for the offense; it is about freeing yourself from the self-imposed anguish it causes you. In *Traveling Mercies* (8), Anne Lamott writes that "not forgiving is like drinking rat poison and then waiting for the rat to die."

Forgiveness is not easy. It can be extremely difficult, but the rewards can be priceless. Forgiving is distinguishing between then and now. Nothing can be done to change then, but now is a choice. Forgiving is a choice—another claim of your rightful power. Forgiving heals the victim, the one who forgives. The *mindful questions* are:

MQ | *What is the motivation for holding on to my bitterness?*

Why am I choosing to burden myself with this grudge when I have the choice of freeing myself of it for good?

Given that I have no control over the offender, what would be the payoff for letting go of my grievance?

BENEFITS OF LETTING GO OF THE PAST

Letting go of the negatives of the past is liberating; it frees us from memories and feelings that only drain energy and fuel discontent. Holding on to discontent is holding on to a stressor that will wear and tear at body and mind.

Not letting go of a negative belief or a belief-driven pattern that is troublesome is like clenching a hot potato in your hand. The pain from the hot potato will get worse, and it will quickly cause tissue damage. Letting go puts an end to a useless and increasingly painful ordeal. Dropping the potato is the only way to cut your losses.

How Does Letting Go
Help Control Diabetes?

Hopefully, you are not weary of seeing this question and getting the same answer. It is so important that it needs to be repeated to make sure you get it. Diabetes care is mostly self-care, and the less stress in your life, the better you will be able to tend to the demands of diabetes. Every stressor that is prevented, eliminated, or minimized spares your body the hardships imposed by the stress response—over the short and long terms. (This might be a good time to go back and review the numerous effects of stress described in Chapters 1 and 2.)

The common beliefs listed on page 182 are more general; the next list is more specific to diabetes.

LET GO OF THESE COMMON, SELF-DEFEATING BELIEFS ABOUT YOU AND DIABETES

- I have to be extremely vigilant and disciplined for good control—often characterized by self-statements that include "always," "never," or other absolute terms.
- I am inferior or less than anyone else because I have diabetes.
- I am destined to suffer serious complications.
- Someone else is responsible for controlling or not controlling my diabetes.
- I am incapable of change.
- Not being able to control my diabetes means I am a failure.
- I have to do something to please someone else, even when doing it is likely to be unhealthy for me.
- I have to have perfect control to avoid complications.
- I have no other choice.
- Everything I think is true.

Acting on any of these beliefs will interfere with your effort to attain and sustain good control of blood glucose levels. Being vigilant is important, but being hypervigilant is likely to be counterproductive. To think that you *always* have to do this or you can *never* do that is wrong and produces stress. The idea that you are destined to suffer serious complications is probably associated with having seen a parent or grandparent endure complications. However, with the medical advances in recent years and with the dramatic increase in knowledge about diabetes control—including the power of stress control—you have many more resources for controlling diabetes than previous generations. Letting go of faulty beliefs frees you of unnecessary burdens as you pursue good glucose control and better health.

BELIEFS THAT OPPOSE LETTING GO

There is a tendency to accept an idea as the truth because it is assumed that the source is indisputable (see Chapter 3: Being Mindful). This bias is especially strong when the source is a family member or someone in a position of power and status. People who belong to an in-group, such as a religious or special interest group, are prone to assume its views are the truth. Going up against the beliefs of any of these sources can fuel fears of conflict, disapproval, and rejection, which is the reason to hold on to these views regardless of the consequences.

Not surprisingly, we are likely to believe and hold on to what fits our established views and interests. It is common for individuals with type 2 diabetes to resist going on insulin because they believe that it means their condition is worsening or that they have failed in controlling diabetes. Individuals who cannot accept the seriousness of diabetes may hold tightly to the belief that it is not a danger to them. Fear about diabetes may be masked by a belief that provides false comfort, at least for a while.

OTHER BARRIERS TO LETTING GO

If a mouse is put into a maze that is designed to provide a pleasant reward when it reaches the end, the mouse will, through trial and error, eventually find its way to the payoff.

Furthermore, the mouse will learn the path to the reward quickly and go there repeatedly—so long as it is rewarded for its effort. However, if, after several successes, the reward is not there, the mouse might try a few more times, but it will give up and stop going there fairly quickly. If a man or woman were put in a similar situation, he or she would find the path to the reward, learn the route, and go there to obtain the prize. But, after having been rewarded several times, when the individual goes to the same place and there is no reward, the individual may still continue to go there time and time again. This person is blinded from reality by the belief that the absence of the prize is the result of some glitch in the system or some statistical matter (think "gambler mentality"). The belief is that the reward will be there the next time, or, if not, the next time after that.

This phenomenon is a theme in Spencer Johnson's *Who Moved My Cheese* (9). Two mice, Hem and Haw, are faced with a dilemma: their previously limitless supply of cheese is gone. Confronted with this dramatic change, each of them reacts differently.

Faced with starving, Haw took the risk of venturing out of his familiar "comfort zone," looking for another source of food. In his search for cheese, Haw had to let go of old beliefs and risk believing differently. At one point in his perilous journey, he said, "The quicker you let go of old cheese, the sooner you find new cheese." Ultimately, he found an abundance of cheese and concluded "old beliefs do not lead you to new cheese."

Sadly, despite the fact that he was starving, Hem rejected Haw's urging to look elsewhere for food. Hem said he liked it where he was. He reasoned, "It's what I know. Besides, it's dangerous out there." Perhaps even more telling, he declared that he was too old to change and too afraid of getting lost to venture from where he was.

The inborn drive to survive draws us to choices that are viewed as safe. Consequently, what is known—what is familiar—is preferred over what is unknown because the former seems to be safer. The comfort of what is familiar can beat the discomfort that it imposes. When Tim has dinner with his family, he eats excessively at their insistence. Avoiding disappointing or displeasing them is more comfortable than the discomfort of confronting their demands. Fear of the unknown often shows itself in "what if" thinking: "What if I fail, what if I make it worse, what if I displease someone, what if I can't stop what I started, or what if I don't like it?"

Letting go often involves taking some risk and may require a degree of self-esteem, confidence, or optimism. Any level of insecurity, such as fear of rejection or abandonment, can make the resistance to letting go insurmountable.

How Can I Develop the Skill of Letting Go?

The process of letting go begins with being mindful of a belief or belief-driven behavior that is working against you. When you become aware of an obstructive belief—which may be apparent as an idea, an attitude, or a feeling that is causing some discomfort or difficulty—the next step is to raise your awareness with a series of *mindful questions*:

MQ | *What belief is driving the discomfort or problem?*

What do I have to let go of to reframe (replace the negative belief with a positive one) in this situation?

Maryjo's interactions with her husband are a continual source of stress. He hovers over her when she is eating and checking her blood glucose, questioning what she is doing, often with a critical tone. Her frustration may escalate to fury, and she often responds in a hostile manner. Their conflicts soar in intensity. Not surprisingly, Maryjo's blood glucose control suffers. She is distracted from what she needs to do and may even be neglecting essential self-care to spite her spouse. Also, the stress from the situation complicates her efforts at control.

Fortunately, Maryjo began to realize that she was in serious trouble and knew that she needed to take control of the situation. She started by asking herself what beliefs were causing her distress. The answer was multilayered. The first faulty belief she identified was concluding that her husband's behavior was proof that he didn't care enough and that, if he cared, he would have understood and trusted her decisions. She assumed that he was disappointed in her for having diabetes. Struggling with the effects of poor glucose control, she concluded that it was his fault and that she was a victim of his hostile behavior. Furthermore, she believed there was no use in trying to get him to work with her to resolve the problem.

A cluster of faulty beliefs was causing her and her husband considerable distress. It was not easy, but with the help of members of a diabetes support group, she was able to let go of the self-defeating beliefs and reframe the problem. The first reframe was that her husband did care a lot about her, and, in fact, his demanding behavior was a result of fears about her health. The only way he was able to express his concerns was to watch closely to see if she was OK. The reframe caused a shift in her feelings from resentment to compassion. The second reframe was to dispute and change the belief that she was a victim of her husband's behavior. She began to understand and accept as the truth that she was responsible for her own care; if there were issues that were impeding her ability to take good care of herself, then she needed to deal with them and not simply assume the posture of a victim. Maryjo realized that feeling that she was the victim was surrendering the power she had to deal with the situation effectively. The positive reframing could not have happened without letting go of her intensely debilitating beliefs.

Letting go usually begins with becoming mindful of a negative feeling or experience. The discontent triggers the process of questioning its cause, which may lead to a frame or behavior that needs to be abandoned. However, you do not have to wait until you are in a jam to practice letting go. When you have some quiet time, use the technique of brainstorming to make a list of frames—beliefs, thoughts, ideas, assumptions—that you are holding on to and that are not working well for you. Start with a persistently distressing endeavor and work backwards to identify the troubling frame.

How Can Brainstorming Help Me Let Go?

Brainstorming is identifying an issue that you want to explore and allowing your mind to roam freely with regard to the issue. It is thinking without restraint. It is asking yourself for solutions to the problem without prejudgments about the value of your thought ("this is silly") or assumptive thinking ("this will never work"). Write down whatever comes to mind. In this process, first reactions are likely to reflect old, well-established ideas. However, brainstorming subsequently surpasses old emotional blocks and old patterns of thinking. Brainstorming is associating with the subject fully and freely. Then, when you have exhausted the possibilities, you can study the list you have accumulated, eliminate the obvious misfits, and look for a potentially winning solution. It is a way of breaking out of conventional and automatic thinking. With regard to letting go, brainstorming might start with a specific issue:

- Control of my diabetes has been a problem, and my doctor has repeatedly suggested that I attend an educational program at a nearby diabetes center. I have repeatedly resisted following his recommendation. What is the problem? What am I resisting? What do I have to let go of to take better care of myself?
- During the week, control of my diabetes is very good. On weekends, it is inconsistent, with serious low or high blood glucose levels occurring frequently. Is there some-

thing I need to let go of to be as consistent on weekends as I am on weekdays?

Brainstorming can also be used to explore possibilities not associated with a specific problem:

- My goal is to reduce the stress caused by beliefs and belief-driven behavior. As I reflect on what is happening at home, at work, and with relationships, what are some beliefs that I might do well to let go of?
- As a single, young adult, dating is a continual source of stress for me. I worry about my date's reaction to my diabetes and about having my blood glucose level drop suddenly. What belief or beliefs are making me anxious when dating?

Letting go is exercising your power by mindfully making the choice to unburden yourself of baggage that weighs heavily on mind and body. Letting go of self-defeating beliefs, behaviors, or grievances is a powerful way of reducing and eliminating unnecessary stress, an enemy of diabetes control.

CHAPTER 10

Winning Frames and Some Losers

Why More Frames?

I t is a fact: choice is power and the more choices, the better. Given that the process of reframing often involves letting go of an ineffective frame and replacing it with a winner, the purpose of this chapter is to present a range of frames that are consistent winners or losers.

Frames to Live By

Operating on faulty frames is one of the major causes of stress. The frame (belief) you put on a situation determines how you think, feel, and behave. A bad frame will have a bad result. Reframing is an ever-present choice for changing an undesirable frame to one that works for you. When you change what you believe about something, you change what it means and you change how it affects you.

Become familiar with these positive frames. Use them often. In living mindfully, you will discover and create many more frames that will enable you to turn undesirable situations into gratifying experiences. When using these frames as a foundation to draw on and to build from, you will have a stress-busting choice for any situation.

Each of these frames can reduce the stress of diabetes and other stressors in your life.

"I Have a Right to Choose What I Believe."

This frame is basic to the practice of reframing. Most of us have a belief system that consists of ideas that we accept as truths but in reality some are not. These "truths" are based on opinions, impressions, and assumptions that have been handed down from generation to generation with no basis in fact. The frame conveys three messages:

- "It is not in my best interest to believe everything I have been led to believe."
- "I am capable of choosing the beliefs that will guide my life."
- "I have that right."

"If I Had Been Where You Have Been, I Would Be Where You Are Now."

This is a frame of compassion for another. When someone is being insensitive or unkind, it is easy to react with anger or by distancing yourself from the offender. Putting yourself in the other person's shoes opens the possibility of coming to an understanding about what the real problem is and, thus, resolving it. In this situation, the *mindful questions* are:

MQ | *What happened to make this person so difficult?*

Can I imagine being in his or her shoes?

What can I do to create a positive outcome?

"Everything is Fascinating!"

Children are fascinated by just about anything. They can be awestruck by the simplest objects and experiences. A child opening a present may be more captivated by the wrapping paper than the present itself. Unfortunately, we lose this wonderful innocence as life becomes very serious too early on. In *The Art of Possibility: Transforming Professional and Personal Life* (10), Ben and Rosamund Stone Zander offer a pathway to regaining that innocence: it is observing our shortcomings and mistakes not as failures or reasons to feel ashamed, but rather with a nonjudgmental curiosity. This frame leads us to see every experience—good or bad—as fascinating, and what is seen as fascinating is never seen as frightening. Can you see having diabetes as fascinating? You know what hypoglycemia or hyperglycemia does, but do you know how the reactions to extreme blood glucose levels happen internally? It is fascinating.

"Maybe?"

I learned this frame from Father Angelo Rizzo, a Catholic priest who devoted his ministry to counseling the mentally disadvantaged. Fr. Rizzo published a monograph of his beliefs in 1980 (11); this frame is one inspiring idea from a brilliant thinker.

Some individuals will stop at almost nothing to win an argument or to defend a position that has no basis in truth. This type of person is determined to be right at any price. Responding to this person's unbending conviction with the frame "maybe?" is accepting that even though you have a different point of view, you are willing to acknowledge that the expressed position "may be" possible. It is a magical way to prevent a senseless argument by agreeing to disagree. Another aspect to this frame is accepting that what we believe "may be" untrue.

"The Best Thing About a Setback Is the Comeback."

This is a quote from Evander Holyfield, who won and lost heavyweight boxing championship titles four times from 1990 to 1994. Common reactions to defeat are an overwhelming sense of failure or shame and the belief that success is impossible. With Mr. Holyfield's frame, a setback becomes an inspiration for making an even bigger and better effort the next time you are challenged. With this frame, a hardship becomes an opportunity.

"I Only Own What Is Mine."

Always taking the blame for whatever goes wrong is a common example of irrational thinking. It is an especially dangerous pattern when someone is prone to blaming you for their discontent. Certainly, if you are at fault, own it. If you have kicked someone in the shin, apologize and make appropriate amends. But if you have done no wrong and you are being accused of something, do not own it. If someone is unjustly throwing darts at you, do not reach out to catch them; give yourself a hug instead.

The fact is that what others do is not because of you. Each of us has a script to play out. The foundation of the script is a system of beliefs, stories, and expectations rooted in those messages from the past or from the pronouncements of those whom we believe to be indisputable.

> *Jane, a 12-year-old with type 1 diabetes, had a severe hypoglycemic episode that caused a dramatic emergency involving a team of paramedics. Jane's mother was very upset. Her reaction was to scold her daughter for being irresponsible. Did Jane cause her mother's grief and punitive behavior? Well, if Jane's blood glucose level had not dropped so low, this event would not have happened. But it is easy to imagine another mother in the same situation reacting very differently, comforting her daughter who has just had a traumatic experience, assuring her that together they will find a solution to the problem that had just occurred. The difference in the reactions of the two mothers is the different scripts by which they live.*

Jane's mother's script is a negative one. It is rooted in a belief system that fuels blame and shame, rampant with irrational "should" and "should nots." Her script reflects what she was taught to believe about herself and life. The other mother's script is positive and optimistic. Her beliefs are about love rather than oriented toward fear. It was Jane's mother's script and not Jane's behavior that determined the antagonistic and unfair reaction. For this situation, the *mindful questions* for Jane's mother to ask are:

MQ | *Jane is a child. Given the challenges of dealing with diabetes and developing interests and desires, how can I react to make such an event an informative experience rather than a confusing and belittling one?*

What can I do when my fears for my daughter fuel intense emotions?

Jane's mom has a problem. It is understandable that she has an emotional reaction when Jane is in danger, but acting out the feelings is harmful to everyone involved. Parents and other caregivers need a plan for "being emotionally smart" (see Chapter 5).

"Taking Care of Myself Is Not Being Selfish."

Doing what is needed to take care of oneself is often confused with being selfish. The clear distinction between the two can be blurred when taking care of oneself disappoints someone else. Have you ever been accused of being selfish when you didn't do what someone wanted you to do? An old saying comes to mind: "The best way to take care of the children is to take care of the mother first." This message applies to everyone—if you take good care of yourself, then you will have what it takes to be there for others. This principle is illustrated by the instructions given to passengers by a flight attendant before commercial airplanes take off. The instruction is that if you have a child with you and it becomes necessary to use the plane's oxygen system, it is essential to put on your oxygen mask first and then put a mask on the child. Obviously, if you passed out from lack of oxygen while trying to put a mask on the child, both you and the child would suffer the consequences. If you are compelled to take care of others to the detriment of your own well-being, the outcome will be unpleasant, if not dangerous.

The frame does not mean that you never make a sacrifice for someone else. It means to make a mindful distinction between being compelled to serve (i.e., to please) someone else as opposed to freely choosing to give up something of yourself in service to someone else who truly needs it.

"No Matter How Rough This Moment Is, There Are Many Reasons to Be Grateful."

Feeling grateful is one of the most positive human feelings. Few emotions are as uplifting physically, mentally, and spiritually. It is easy to get stuck in negative thinking, to dwell on one's misfortune. But even in the worst of circumstances, there are reasons to be grateful. Choosing to change your focus from what is wrong or bad to what is right or good is taking control of how you think and feel, which is the power of *mindfulness*. Refer back to pages 148–152 for tips on how to be grateful.

"It Is OK to Feel This Way, But I Do Not Have to Act on It Mindlessly."

Feelings are never wrong. They simply are what they are. What is wrong is acting on a feeling impulsively or compulsively, which, in either case, is likely to have a bad outcome. Because most of our values and beliefs are well established at an early age, you did not have the chance to choose what you do and do not believe. Many of the beliefs you acquired are likely to be highly charged emotionally. Consequently, feelings emerge automatically, not by choice. Being cut off by the driver ahead of you may trigger a strong desire to catch up with him to tell him off.

It is not wrong to be annoyed; however, it would be very wrong to act on the feeling. Instead, by being emotionally smart (see Chapter 5), you recognize and accept the feeling and make a well-informed choice about what to do.

> Brad had suffered through several years of poor glucose control, but he was able to reverse the situation and get good control of his diabetes. He was taking good care of himself. At a family party, his older brother, Tom, kept insisting that Brad eat various foods that he did not want to eat. The more Brad refused, the more persistent Tom became, despite knowing of Brad's intense effort to achieve good control of his blood glucose levels. Brad was angry and struggled to resist cursing at Tom or throwing the food right into his brother's face.

Brad's feelings are understandable, but acting on them would have been a big mistake. Mindfully applying this frame of acceptance and self-control, Brad thanked Tom for wanting him to have the treats. He explained that trying to force him to eat something he did not want was not helpful. He told Tom that it would be very helpful if he trusted and supported his choices, since he was doing so well in controlling his diabetes. Eliciting Tom's help got through to his brother. Tom got the message. If Brad's reaction to Tom's aggressiveness had been quarrelsome, the outcome would have been unpleasant for both of them.

"The Precious Present Is the Best Place to Be."

Participants in Alcoholics Anonymous are told that there are 2 days of the week they should never have to worry about— yesterday and tomorrow. The reason should be obvious: there is nothing that can be done about either one. Yesterday cannot be changed, and nothing can be done today about tomorrow. The only time we have the power to control our destiny is in the precious present.

Have you ever had a medical procedure or a high-stakes meeting scheduled for some time in the future and you worried about it for days or even weeks? The fear aroused in anticipation of an event can be worse than the event itself. Imagining the worst that can happen and filling your mind with "what if this, what if that" causes the same distress that would occur if this or that actually happened. All of that suffering is due to not being in the moment. Being in the present keeps the past and future completely neutralized.

Certainly there are times when referring to the past or future is sensible. Past experiences can provide valuable lessons about what to do or what not to do in the present, and planning for the future is important. The key is whether being in the past or future is a mindful activity. Mindlessly drifting to another time than the present is at the very least wasteful, and it can be costly.

"A Good Feeling Is Only One Thought Away."

This frame (attributed to psychologist Sheila Krystal) is a reminder that you can choose to stay in a negative place or choose to change the way you are thinking about the immediate situation so that you are able to change the way you feel. Changing the frame or the imagery that is dragging you down is always a possibility.

> *Karson goofed up. She will occasionally have an alcoholic beverage at a social event, but it is usually a single drink. However, at a party with friends, she had several drinks, which lessened her inhibitions and led to eating a lot of junk food. Later, with a hangover and a blood glucose level of 350 mg/dL, she began to torment herself with self-demeaning thoughts: "I am weak. I am stupid. My behavior was shameful." With each self-criticism, Karson felt worse. But she was able to mindfully reflect on how well she does most of the time in taking care of herself. Smiling, she said, "I may not be perfect, but some of me is wonderful." This thought, with a touch of humor, felt good and enabled her to get past the mistake she had made at the party.*

"I Mindfully Reject the Temptation to Act on an Assumption."

When we assume something, we accept that it is true without checking or confirming it. It is taken for granted to be real. A wrong assumption can be relatively harmless: "I assume my spouse knows what I want for my birthday." But an assumption can also be stressful or dangerous. Thinking "I am feeling low, but I'm only 20 minutes from home, so I'll wait until I get there to check my blood glucose" assumes you are only a short while from being home with nothing in your way. But what if there has been a traffic accident on the way and now you are 2 hours from home? Acting on an assumption is acting mindlessly; it is operating on automatic pilot. When the stakes are high, it is essential to be more cautious and to check the validity of an assumption. Regardless of the stakes, it is always wise to resist the tendency to act on an assumption and to act on as much information as possible instead. When in the slightest doubt, put the assumption to the test:

MQ | *What evidence is there to support the truth of this assumption?*

Obviously, there are assumptions that we live by that are almost certain to be true, such as driving through an intersection when we have a green light, assuming drivers that have the red light will stop, or taking a medication or having surgery because we assume that the doctor knows what is best for us.

"I Intend to Have a Nifty Day Today."

Holding on to an irrational fear can spoil even the best days. The feeling of fear does not have to be based on anything real. If you believe that something will harm you, mind and body will react as if the threat is real, causing you anxiety and stress. The NIFTY (**N**o **I**rrational **F**ears **T**oda**Y**) frame reminds you to identify your irrational fears and to vow that you will not let them spoil your day. You have that choice.

Each of these frames is a consistent winner. Use them for reframing situations that have been causing you distress. As you use these frames more and more, you will find yourself discovering and creating other winning frames that work for your own unique circumstances and needs.

LOSING FRAMES

If you were traveling to a country that you knew very little about, would you seek information that would guide your decisions about the trip? It would be important to know where to go and what (if anything) to avoid. Similarly, in life and the journey of diabetes management, it is as vital to know what not to do as it is to know what to do.

The frames presented in this section deserve special attention because each one is a troublemaker. Being mindful of them will prevent you from becoming their victim.

**"If I Manage My Diabetes Perfectly,
I Will Not Have Any Problems With the Diabetes."**

If you could do everything perfectly, you might expect to have total control of your diabetes. There are two problems with this reasoning. First, perfection is impossible. No one is perfect. No one is without flaws or faults, and we cannot totally avoid mistakes. Second, what you do may not be all that is affecting your blood glucose level. You may be well disciplined and think your behavior was *exactly* the same on two consecutive days, but there was an unexpected spike in your blood glucose level. Perhaps there are other physiological factors involved (illness or hormones, for example) or you heard a vague comment at work that was stressful. There are numerous, subtle stimuli in everyone's life that can have unexpected consequences. In fact, it is possible to have unconscious fear-related memories that can have a dramatic effect on everyday behavior and emotions.

*James, a 65-year-old man, came to the Johns Hopkins
Comprehensive Diabetes Center with late-onset type 2*

diabetes. He was aware of the possible complications associated with diabetes, and he was determined to prevent any serious problems by practicing his version of perfect self-care. James decided that perfect diabetes manage-ment meant maintaining blood glucose levels in the range of 95–105 mg/dL, and he checked his blood glucose every waking hour to be sure he was in his self-defined zone. This meant sticking himself about 16 times a day, which had to be hard on his skin, but more important, each time he checked his blood glucose was stressful. James believed that it was necessary to maintain extremely tight control. He was anxious to have his blood glucose levels fall into the designated range. Waiting each time for the meter to calculate the blood glucose level was tense. Would it be in the needed range? What if it wasn't? When his blood glucose level wasn't in the desired range, which was often, James was filled with doom and despair. His belief that perfection was the answer to his fears was completely counter to what he wanted to accomplish.

Striving to attain your personal best is the ideal goal. The frame of being perfect is setting the perfect trap for failure. A frame that positively addresses the issue of perfection is, "When I do my personal best, I am in the best place possible."

"If I Bury My Head in the Sand, the Problem Will Go Away."

Denying the seriousness of a situation is dangerous. However unpleasant or scary the circumstances may be, the best chance you have of coming out on top is to face the music as soon as possible. Denial will delay facing a problem, but only in the short term. Ultimately, the problem will prevail or worsen, and you will be forced to deal with it. Also, a delay is likely to make resolving the problem more difficult physically and mentally. Try this frame if you are tempted to bury your head in the sand: "However scary it is, I am better off knowing and dealing with it now."

"She Should, He Ought To, They Have To . . . Then I Will Be Happy."

Any frame with "should," "ought to," or "have to" is probably a trap. The belief that someone has to do what you expect for you to be happy is rooted in the conviction that you are a victim of that person's actions. The "victim stance" is a relentless stress-producing machine. It is all right to want someone to change, but expecting that person to change is an invitation for trouble. Depending on others for your happiness is giving power to someone else. It is surrendering control to another. Accepting responsibility for your own happiness is claiming your power and taking control of your destiny.

If you get trapped into blaming someone for your unhappiness, try this frame: "Contentment is an inside job, and I whole-heartedly accept responsibility for my happiness."

"I'm Not Enough!"

Anyone who was raised in a dysfunctional environment is likely to be haunted by this demeaning self-assessment. Children who experience the dissatisfaction of a parent or any other authority figure will interpret the criticism as a personal failure. Not being able to meet the expectations of a parent or teacher—however unreasonable—leads the child to conclude that he or she is defective or too flawed to satisfy anyone. Believing you are not enough leads to trying desperately to be enough, to do whatever it takes to please others, regardless of the emotional cost. It means doing everything possible to get the approval of others, even if it causes self-suffering. This frame invites other self-defeating beliefs: "I have to put everyone else's needs ahead of my own," "I have to prove I am OK," and "If I am perfect, I will get their approval." Any of these frames can be very stressful and detrimental to managing diabetes and living a quality life.

Use these frames when you are feeling that you are not enough: "There will be moments when I am not enough, but in the big picture, I am enough and more" or "I may not be perfect, but some of my parts are beautiful."

"It Could Not Be Worse. I Can't Stand It. I Give Up."

The bad news is that people believe these words and suffer the uncomfortable feelings that accompany them. The good news is that none of the parts of this frame are likely to be true. First, aside from the most extreme circumstances, whatever you are experiencing could be worse. Second, you are able to stand it or you wouldn't be talking about it. Last, you have not given up. You may be momentarily overwhelmed, but you can keep going. The key is to stop obsessing about what is not working—including this frame—and adopting a winning frame and a mindful plan for success.

"For Me, It Has to Be All or Nothing."

You may recognize this frame by a story that everyone has heard.

> Debra needs to lose weight because her obesity is hindering her ability to manage her diabetes. She has a plan and gets off to a good start. For two and a half weeks, she followed her plan exactly and lost 9 pounds. In the middle of the third week, Debra went to a family gathering known for its array of homemade treats. Although she did not eat everything in sight, she did eat considerably more than her plan allowed. Her response: she stopped her weight loss program, returning to her old pattern of consuming excessive calories. For Debra, it was "all or nothing." Her expectations were rigid and inflexible. Having struck out in the third inning, she believed she had lost and quit the game.

This frame is extremely limiting. There is no room for adjustment. With an "all or nothing" point of view, it is impossible to see the positive elements in a situation. Debra had exercised good control for 16 of 17 days, and she had lost 9 pounds. But because she had not done "all" of what she had intended, she concluded "nothing" had been done.

Here is a frame that will help you overcome the faulty belief in "all or nothing": "I want to achieve it all, but I am grateful for what I can accomplish, so long as I have given my best effort."

"Change Is Too Risky."

You may never have consciously thought these words, but chances are you have lived them. It is easy to find a reason for backing off from making a change—not enough time to deal with that right now, not believing it would make a difference, etc. The likely reason, however, is that the anticipation of changing something that is so familiar is scary. We tend to hold on to what is familiar because, as strange as it may be, it is comfortable, even though it may actually be quite unsettling. We don't do well with uncertainty, and there is a certainty to what is familiar, even if it causes us hardship. When what you are doing over and over again is having a negative effect on you and you do not make the changes necessary to end your dismay, you are surrendering your power to the fear of change.

The fear of uncertainty exaggerates the sense of risk in change. Mindfully challenging the reality of the risk and comparing the genuine threat with the potential reward will help you overcome this barrier. If change is consistently difficult for you, consider the words of Ralph Waldo Emerson: "He has not learned the lesson of life who does not every day surmount a fear." More recently, author Erica Jong has said: "I have accepted fear as a part of life, specifically the fear of change . . . I have gone ahead despite the pounding in the heart that says: turn back."

With the messages of Emerson and Jong in mind, here is a frame to use when taking a reasonable risk is blocked by unsupported fear: "For me to take a risk does not require the absence of fear; it insists on the presence of courage."

"I Don't Have the Time to Do All of This."

In this modern world, this frame is as common as apple pie. The need for more and to have it faster drives us to do more and at higher speeds. Although the rewards may be desirable, the overall picture can be quite the opposite. Living in the fast lane drains one's energy and thus one's effectiveness. Multitasking takes attention away from other important issues. Only so much can be done at one time. The essentials of self-care may be overlooked, including adequate rest, sleep, exercise, play, and attention to the details of diabetes management. Making a mindful assessment of what you are doing will distinguish between what is necessary and what is not. Begin by ranking activities in order of importance and dropping what is not essential. Eliminating excess baggage is a great way to simplify each and every day.

Are There Other Frames to Avoid?

Given that a frame is a consequence of the interaction between an individual's beliefs and the situation at hand, it might take a few volumes to cover the frames not considered in this chapter—both frames to avoid and frames to draw on regularly.

HOW CAN I IDENTIFY THE FRAMES THAT I NEED TO TRASH?

Jot down the issues and circumstances that are consistently causing you stress. Then, for each disturbing situation you listed, ask these *mindful questions*:

MQ | *What frames (beliefs, assumptions, attitudes) are involved in this problem?*

Which of these frames are causing the distress?

Is there a sensible reason for not trashing this troubling frame?

Make a list of each frame you have identified as distressing, and carry the list with you as a warning to avoid giving them any credibility. It is as important to avoid doing what is wrong as it is to choose doing what is right. Every disarmed booby trap is a huge win.

CHAPTER 11

Problem Solving

Why Is Problem Solving Important?

Problems are inevitable. Some are small, and some are big, but no one escapes dealing with issues that need to be resolved. For some, the journey of life might be described as passage from one problem to the next. As you know, diabetes can generate a range of challenges. There are real problems and imaginary ones, but whether real or imagined, the effects are real. And when a problem is not solved, the consequences can be very stressful and even dangerous.

Problem solving, particularly in the Western world, tends to be an impulsive act. We are conditioned to fix it right away, to make the problem go away. Call your doctor and describe the symptoms you are having, and you are likely to have medication quickly prescribed—without being examined. This approach may work in the short term but won't be beneficial over time. The way to consistently and effectively work out problems is to have a mindful, informed approach for resolving issues.

Being an effective problem-solver is an important objective for anyone with diabetes. It is a powerful tool for addressing matters that might otherwise impede the ability to either negate stress or manage the disease.

Although some problems require an immediate response, most are solved effectively by an orderly process that is rooted in being mindful. A detailed model for solving problems will be covered, but first let's look at some conditions that typically become problematic.

What Are Some of the Common Causes of Problems?

By now you may have an answer to the question above: mindlessly acting on faulty frames (beliefs). Responding to troublesome circumstances with a frame that says "I can't," "I'm not good enough," "I'm just unlucky," "I give up," "I am a helpless victim," or some other form of self-defeating resignation will not only cause problems but also make it improbable that they can be solved. Here are some other common conditions that will create problems:

- Staying attached to ideas, objects, and behaviors that do not work for you (not being able to let go).
- Having unrealistic expectations of self and others (look for frames that include "should," "have to," or "must").
- Allowing a "want" to become a "need."
- Clinging to grudges and grievances.
- Denying responsibility (playing the victim and blaming others).
- Being inappropriately responsible (remember the winning frame from Chapter 10: "I Only Own What Is Mine").
- Treating stories as facts.
- Giving in to an irrational fear.
- Acting on impulse, whim, or feeling.
- Acting on assumptions.

The means for overcoming each of these troublemakers are presented in various ways throughout the book. Applying the model that follows is an effective approach for solving most problems.

A Model for Solving Problems

STEP 1. RECOGNIZE THERE IS A PROBLEM

Awareness of a problem is usually triggered by feelings. When faced with an undesirable predicament, we are likely to feel worried, sad, anxious, frustrated, or even very angry, any of which are reliable signals that a problem exists. Recognizing that there is a problem may also come from the words or actions of another. Recognizing that there is a problem is usually not an issue. However, it is possible to be in trouble and not believe there is a problem or that it is someone else's burden to bear. If you are experiencing any discomfort that persists, the *mindful questions* are:

MQ | *Are my thoughts, my feelings, or the messages I'm receiving from others telling me that I have a problem?*

Is there a problem that I need to attend to?

STEP 2. STOP. TAKE A FEW BREATHS

Acting on emotions, which is common, or acting mindlessly (automatically, impulsively, compulsively, or habitually) is likely to make a problem intractable or even worsen the situation. Therefore, the next step in solving a problem is to pause and take a deep breath, which opens the possibility of a mindful approach to resolving an undesirable situation. The more serious the matter, the more important the pause becomes.

The pause may be very brief. There are circumstances that demand a quick reaction, such as becoming aware that your blood glucose level is getting too low. If the situation is urgent, then you will have to act quickly. But generally taking a pause is an effective step in solving problems.

A mantra or brief meditation can be an excellent way to enhance the pause. When this thought came to me, I wrote this haiku poem:

Just another bump
One more obstacle to jump
Done with room to spare

In Chapter 7: Choosing the Style in Lifestyle, you were encouraged to make creativity a part of your way of living. I write haiku poetry to pause and relax and, sometimes, to get a different angle on things. In this example, my purpose is to put problems into perspective, that is, to not take everything so seriously and to not "make a mountain out of a molehill."

STEP 3. DEFINE THE PROBLEM

Problems are uncomfortable, and you may have a tendency to do something quickly to fix them, which can be a mistake. Unless immediate action is necessary, a good solution to a problem is likely to come when the issues are identified and clearly understood. The *mindful questions* are:

MQ | *What is the problem? (Strive for an answer that is as specific and precise as possible.)*

What issues are contributing to the problem?

Does this problem call for reframing a faulty belief?

These questions are not likely to be a surprise, but answering them is not always simple. People with diabetes frequently have problems with the significant people in their lives nagging about what they eat. The definition of this problem needs to be as specific as possible to be useful. The underlying problem that needs to be addressed may be that the person receiving the complaint is indeed eating poorly and, thus, scaring the nagger, who is anxious and desperately trying to get the person with diabetes to change behaviors. It may be that the significant other lacks adequate knowledge about diabetes self-care and is reacting inappropriately. It certainly could be a combination of both circumstances. Here are some *mindful questions* to get to the core of a problem:

MQ	*What circumstances are present when the problem occurs?*
	When this problem occurs, is anyone else involved?
	Is it always the same person or people? Is there a pattern to this problem?
	Am I a part of the problem? If so, how?

Looking back at the problem of being nagged about what you eat, you may, in this process of self-questioning, realize that only one person is involved with this issue. It might become apparent that this individual is overreacting because he or she has a limited, outdated perspective on diabetes. With a lack of knowledge or by acting on misinformation, your behavior has been perceived as improper, even inept. If you simply accept the criticism without reflection, there is a problem with potentially serious consequences. Keep in mind that some people still believe that people with diabetes cannot eat anything that contains sugar. I have heard diabetes referred to as the "sugar disease" many times. So part of the solution to the problem is to inform this person about some of the facts of good diabetes care. In answering the series of questions, you may also realize that because the nagging has irritated you, you have reacted with resentment, which has heightened the conflict. Instead

Problem Solving

of trying to communicate information that might ease this concern, you show your irritation, which leaves both of you uncomfortable and the matter unresolved. So another part of the solution is to be aware of and control your emotional reaction to the nagging. Also, if your frame for the situation is that she "should understand," then that in itself is part of the problem, and reframing is part of the solution. A mindful frame would be that, "I need to try to educate her about eating and diabetes." The key to this part of the model is to be as specific as possible in defining the problem.

STEP 4. REFLECT ON POSSIBLE SOLUTIONS

This is the time when you think about what choices are available for solving the problem. This process is similar to that of setting and achieving a goal (see Chapter 4). To start, the *mindful question* is:

> *MQ* | *What barriers stand in the way of solving the problem?*

You probably have heard the old saying, "Know thine enemy." The clearer you are about what you are up against, the better your chance of coming out on top. Here are some common deterrents to solving a problem.

- *Being locked on a detail and missing the big picture.* It would be a sad mistake to avoid a loving aunt or friend because she nags you from time to time about what you are eating.
- *Being locked on "you," not "me."* In solving a problem between two or more people, it is essential to identify what role you play in it. Taking the role of victim will only make the situation worse and unsolvable.
- *Missing the opportunity to get the advice of reliable and worthy others.* The input from others, especially anyone who is familiar with or affected by the problem, can be very helpful. There is no shame in asking for help; the shame is in not asking.

- *Lacking—or not using—the problem-solving skills described in this chapter.* If, for example, you do not define the problem clearly or fail to pause to reflect on the issues involved, you will have made finding a solution very difficult, if not impossible.

Also, review the conditions that commonly cause problems listed earlier in this chapter. Conditions that cause difficulties are often the same forces that keep the undesirable situation alive.

After you have reflected on and identified the barriers to successful resolution of a problem, the next *mindful questions* are:

| *MQ* | *What strengths and resources do I have to solve the problem?* |
| | *Will what has worked for me in the past help me in this situation?* |

In Chapter 12 on page 231, there is an exercise to help you identify your current and potential strengths. Everyone has a treasure chest of strengths, although many lose sight of them for one reason or another. It is essential to achieving the best possible management of stress, diabetes, and life to know your strengths—to build on them and develop new ones. Here are some general guidelines, but if you have not done the exercise in Chapter 12, please do it as soon as possible.

- Whatever you are good at is a strength.
- Anyone in your support network who has the ability to help solve the problem can be a source of strength for you.
- What you have used to succeed in other situations may be helpful in solving the current problem.
- If you are stuck, there is a lesson in this book that will help you move forward. Find it and put it to work for you.

At this point, the *mindful questions* are:

MQ | *What are the possibilities for solving this problem?*

As I work through this model, what choices are emerging for solving the problem?

Would brainstorming be helpful at this time?
(See page 190.)

Several times in this book, you are urged to make a list of what comes to mind. This is another such time. In this case, write down some of what you have come up with in this step. Develop an index of strengths and resources in one corner and barriers to solving the problem in another spot. Next, list the solutions that come to mind with this information in front of you. With all of the issues and possibilities there in front of you, the pieces of the puzzle will begin to come together.

If you are still not satisfied that you have found a good approach to the problem, you can begin a "brainstorming" exercise. Again, this works best by writing down your thoughts. Brainstorming is letting your mind go free, searching for possibilities without restraint. It is asking yourself for solutions to the problem without the restraints of prejudgments ("this is stupid") or assumptive thinking ("the other party won't like this idea"). In the process of searching for solutions to a problem, first reactions are likely to reflect old beliefs; brainstorming subsequently surpasses old emotional blocks and old patterns of thinking. Brainstorming is associating with the subject fully and freely. Then, when you have exhausted the possibilities, you can study the list, eliminate the obvious misfits, and look for a potentially winning solution.

If, after applying these reflective techniques, a solution to the problem is not apparent, the next *mindful question* is:

MQ | *Is the problem so complex that it requires an incremental approach?*

If a problem has several parts, it can quickly become overwhelming. This situation requires the opposite approach to seeing the big picture. It requires breaking down the problem into smaller elements and tackling the parts one by one.

> *Marc is overweight and depressed, and his blood glucose level is usually in the range of 250–350 mg/dL. His doctor told him he had to change his eating habits, exercise regularly, and see someone for his depression. It was all too much for Marc to deal with at the same time; consequently, he did nothing. Marc needs to break his predicament into three separate problems: diet, exercise, and depression. Because his depression is likely to be affecting the other issues, it probably should be the first matter he addresses. When he is able to get the depression under control, he will be able to address one of the other problems.*

Addressing one problem at a time—or each aspect of a multilevel problem separately—will make meeting the challenge more manageable.

STEP 5. CHOOSE THE BEST APPROACH FOR SOLVING THE PROBLEM AND DO IT

Every problem will not require the detailed analysis described above; but when it is used, you will arrive at a sound answer to the problem at hand. If you have done the steps and are still doubtful, ask these *mindful questions*:

MQ | *What is the frame that is keeping me from moving forward?*

> *Is it typical for me to procrastinate, to always assume that there must be a better way?*

There is almost always some degree of uncertainty and risk when acting to solve a problem. There comes a time to take the risk and do it.

STEP 6. EXERCISE YOUR CHOSEN SOLUTION MINDFULLY, EVALUATING THE RESULTS AND MAKING ADJUSTMENTS ACCORDINGLY

Throughout your effort to solve the problem, the **mindful questions** are:

MQ
> *Is my approach to this problem working?*
>
> *If it is not working, what do I need to do to make it work?*

Once you have a game plan, it makes no sense to follow it mindlessly, regardless of how sound it appeared at the start. It is essential to gauge the results of your actions and make adjustments as needed.

There may be times when it is necessary to go back to the beginning of the problem-solving model and start again. If this happens, it is very important to pay attention to the frame you put around it. For some, it can be very easy to take on the frame of failure. A more appropriate and useful frame would be, "This has been an opportunity to learn about myself and the process of problem solving, and I will succeed in solving this problem."

The Problem-Solving Model in Action

Jeff's job often requires urgent and prolonged attention. At these times, it is impossible to maintain his regular self-care routine. Jeff has had several distressing episodes of hypoglycemia because he was distracted by these work-related emergencies.

After a few false-starts, Jeff was able to define the problem as a lack of preparation on his part. Despite the fact that the problem had occurred several times, he did not have a self-care plan for the times when his regular routine was disrupted. Jeff had a very responsible job because he was good at reflecting mindfully to get to the root of the problem, thereby, eliminating the problem. He used this same mindful approach to resolve the problem of being distracted from essential self-care in the workplace. He obtained a continuous glucose monitoring device that provides continuous, real-time readings and sends alerts when preset levels are breached or trending toward unwanted levels. In addition, he carries glucose tablets and a snack pack with him at all times so he can quickly absorb glucose when he begins to feel low. Also, Jeff informed two men—who are usually with him on these urgent assignments—about the symptoms of hypoglycemia, a move that gave him added protection. By asking the *mindful questions* (see above) leading to sound problem-solving techniques, Jeff eliminated the likelihood of a bad episode of hypoglycemia on the job. He identified the problem, his strengths, and the resources available to solve it.

Jocelyn has the opportunity to travel in Europe for several weeks, but she is on insulin, and the invitation is a dilemma for her. Having diabetes, she has always felt vulnerable and has approached self-care conservatively. Thinking of taking the trip is stressful. She is concerned about how she can take syringes on a plane with the strict regulations imposed at airports and how she will replenish her insulin supply in a foreign land, when needed.

Jocelyn's travel companions made her aware that she was making the problem bigger than it was by ruminating on worst-case scenarios. Challenged by her friends, she was able to shift into a problem-solving mode. Jocelyn recognized that the problem and solution were multilayered. First, she had made assumptions without getting the facts about traveling with insulin-treated diabetes. She contacted the airline and learned that she could take her insulin supplies aboard the plane. She decided she would take enough insulin for twice the length of time she would be away, and she would take backup basal and bolus insulin in pen form for extra protection. She learned, too, that she could see a physician in the country she was visiting and get a prescription for insulin if necessary. Also, she realized she had other valuable resources: her two friends were very dependable, caring women. She would not be alone. They would be a constant source of support and strength. In addition to giving herself the treat of a trip to Europe, overcoming her apprehensions boosted her self-esteem. She was proud of her ability to overcome an old problem that had deprived her of traveling outside the country in the past. With the support of her friends, Jocelyn found a solution to each element of her multilayered problem.

> *David, a teen with type 1 diabetes, had not had many dates. He was self-conscious about diabetes and chose to avoid dating. But he met Jill, whom he really liked, and he found the courage to ask her out. He was excited that she had said yes, but he quickly became uneasy about telling her that he had diabetes. David began the process of defining the problem by reviewing the pros and cons of revealing or concealing his medical condition.*
>
> *If David told Jill he had diabetes, then she might think he is flawed or undesirable and change her mind about going out with him. Or she might be unnerved at the prospect of being with someone with a condition she knows nothing about. Not revealing that he had diabetes would relieve his concerns about being rejected so long as nothing*

went wrong on the date. It would be essential to prevent an episode of hypoglycemia or an extreme rise in blood glucose level, but he would not be able to check his blood glucose or openly inject insulin. What if the evening did not go the way he expected, and his blood glucose level began to fall or it soared and he needed insulin? Just having it on his mind would be stressful. Because he is an honest and caring person, he knew he would feel guilty for starting a relationship with a secret.

Using the problem-solving model, David realized that the problem was internal and that he had created a pessimistic scenario without a clue as to how Jill would respond to his condition. He realized, too, that one of his strengths was his compassion and that he was very considerate of others. It also occurred to him that he was attracted to Jill in part because of her sensitivity and caring nature. Then, he imagined reversing roles. How would he react if on their first date she revealed that she had diabetes? He envisioned that he would be very supportive, asking questions about diabetes so that he could understand what it was like for her to have this burden. He knew he would ask her what they needed to do to make the date safe for her. Imagining the relationship in reverse, he felt confident that the best solution to his problem was to tell her he had diabetes and inform her of the details that would make it comfortable for both of them.

This example illustrates an important point in the process of problem solving: what might initially appear as the cause of the problem may not be so. It would have been easy for David to blame his diabetes for the problem or simply to make assumptions about Jill, which in effect would have put the blame on her. Fortunately, he was able to resist a shallow definition of the matter and conclude that the defining issue was an uninformed picture he had created about how she would react to his medical condition.

Angie loves to jog. It helps her manage her weight and blood glucose levels. The problem was that she really wanted to run a marathon, which she assumed was not possible because of her diabetes. The main concern was the possibility that her blood glucose level would drop dangerously low, but imagining stopping several times over the more than 26-mile race to check her blood glucose was emotionally overpowering. She knew that others with diabetes had run endurance races, including triathlon events, but these runners had required the assistance of medical teams to help maintain in-range glucose levels. When friends ran a marathon or even when she knew about a marathon that was taking place, she felt frustrated and depressed. This was the one diabetes-related issue that really got her into a bad emotional state.

One day, after reading about someone who had overcome extreme odds to achieve a lifelong dream, Angie was inspired to pursue her own dream with renewed determination. Although she was not familiar with the problem-solving model, she applied its principles quite naturally (it is, after all, a very common sense process). Angie realized that she had given up on her dream because she assumed it couldn't be done without having an extensive support system, which was not practical to consider. Having made the assumption, she never thought about the possibility of another way to run the marathon. Believing it could not be done was the cause of the problem and the barrier to its solution.

Determined to pursue every possibility, Angie turned to the local diabetes clinic and discussed the matter with a certified diabetes educator. This professional care provider became a dynamic resource for Angie. She advised Angie of technological advances that she could use to make the long run possible. She informed Angie of the continuous glucose monitoring system, which measures interstitial fluid glucose levels. The device measures blood glucose levels every few minutes and signals significant changes in glucose levels as well as readings that exceed preset limits. Knowing that her blood glucose level was dropping would signal her to drink fortified fluids to bring the level back into the normal range. Knowing that the system would signal her if her blood glucose level exceeded the preset "safe" range eliminated the risk that she would suffer hypoglycemia during the event. To further ensure a safe and successful marathon, she would maintain a cell phone link with the diabetes educator. Angie also asked her friends to stand along the course to provide necessary fluids and moral support. Angie solved the problem and will run the marathon with confidence and enthusiasm.

An unsolved problem is a source of unending stress. Unfortunately, many problems are either never solved or are acted on mindlessly, with unfavorable consequences. The surest way to solve a problem is to use a deliberate, informed approach, taking into consideration each element of the problem and its solution. The model presented in this chapter provides an effective tool for making problems an opportunity to turn difficult circumstances into advantages. When a problem is thoroughly analyzed, it not only might lead to a solution, but may also result in other benefits. In Angie's story, she not only solved the problem of managing her diabetes while running a marathon but also—in learning of the continuous glucose monitoring system—eliminated another diabetes-related hardship. Now, using the continuous monitoring system, she will no longer be blindsided by a dramatic change in glucose levels—not even in her sleep.

In each example, the power of mindful problem solving is obvious: stress is eliminated, and opportunity is seized.

CHAPTER 12

Anticipate It

How Will Anticipation Help Manage Diabetes?

Stressors, the sources of the stress response, are often repetitive. They occur time and time again. Everyone has routines, patterns of behavior, and things we do the same way and usually at the same time of the week or month. Everyone does some things by habit. The problem is that even when these customary activities do not work well and cause stress, they are so ordinary that we simply do not recognize either the flawed patterns or the opportunity to learn from them. This behavior is repeated over and over, and we get stressed again and again. The next time the situation occurs, we do the same thing with the same outcome. If the outcome is stressful, then it will be a source of distress every time.

If a situation is likely to occur again with the same undesirable consequences, then there is an opportunity to do something different that will cause something different to happen—something different and better. Doing the same thing again and again, despite the fact that what you are doing doesn't work, is throwing control out the window. By anticipating the likelihood of a bad outcome, you are taking the first step in controlling what happens.

Once again, being mindful saves the day. When you pay attention to what happens, to what works or does not work, you can avoid the pitfalls that tripped you in the past. Foreseeing the potential for an undesirable situation enables you to do something to avoid repeating it. Anticipating and eliminating a stressful situation is taking control; it is claiming the power that is rightfully yours. The more you are in control, the less stress you will experience and the more successful your diabetes management will be.

How Can I Develop This Skill?

Here are some ways to develop your ability for anticipating and eliminating stressors that have repeatedly troubled you. The *mindful question* is:

> MQ | *What do I do over and over again, with the same undesirable results?*

1. *Use your memory to your advantage.* This is a time to mindfully scan the past. If you are going to a family picnic, what happened when you went last time? Were you unable to resist Aunt Jane's incredible chocolate cheesecake or the fried chicken and barbecued ribs waiting to be devoured? If your last experience was not good, then that is the signal. With that memory, you have anticipated the probability of a stressful situation. Sometimes the memory is not conscious, but your body is responding to the threat, in which case you may feel uneasy when you think about going to the picnic but not know exactly why. Remember from Chapter 8: Reframing, that any physical or emotional discomfort is a signal to pay attention, a signal that something is not right. The *mindful questions* are:

> MQ | *Is there anything about an upcoming event to which I should pay special attention?*
>
> *Is the discomfort I am feeling about the upcoming event telling me something?*

2. *Create a vulnerabilities list.* Knowing what you are vulnerable to is the first step in eliminating it. A vulnerability is a situation that puts you at risk of a bad experience. Make a list of the situations that are likely to cause you to feel stressed. It is important to write them down because the process of writing raises the information to a higher level of awareness, which is essential to using this powerful aspect of mindfulness. The **mindful question** is:

MQ | *What situations repeatedly cause me grief?*

Some common examples of vulnerability are:
- "Every time I go to happy hour with my coworkers, I eat and drink too much, and I end up feeling physically ill and bad about myself."
- "All of our social events are centered on eating, and neither diabetes nor heart-healthy dishes are considered for these gatherings."
- "What frightens me most about having diabetes is hypoglycemia. My mother has passed out several times when her blood glucose level dropped too low, and I have come close several times because. . . ."
- "I forget to do what is necessary to manage my blood glucose level (such as checking my blood glucose, taking my medications, or eating sensibly), especially on holidays and vacations."
- "When I am eating and someone questions what I am eating because I have diabetes, I get very angry. It feels as if they are accusing me of being irresponsible or stupid."

Identifying what triggers strong emotional reactions will enable you to manage your vulnerabilities effectively. Overreacting emotionally can be stressful or lead to behavior that becomes stressful (see Chapter 5: Being Emotionally Smart).

3. *Find or create alternatives for the situations that make you vulnerable.* Choice is power. Once you identify your vulnerabilities, you have the opportunity to make choices

that save you from falling back into situations that have been unfavorable before. Mindfully exercising choices gives you the ability to avoid common stressors, thereby increasing your physical and emotional wellness—a wellness that helps your diabetes management efforts. The *mindful questions* are:

MQ | *Given the circumstances, what changes can I make that will work for me?*

Given my vulnerability at these events, is my best choice to skip it?

Some examples of alternatives to situations that are common for many with diabetes are:

- I like to join my coworkers after work for happy hour as an opportunity to bond with them, which is important to me. The problem is that these events lead to overeating and drinking, which is not what I want to do. So I started inviting coworkers to my home, where I serve light fare and we socialize by playing games. Enjoying these activities together really is a better way of bonding.

- Instead of having food at the center of a social event, have a gathering where the focus is on mirth and humor. Have light snacks, but instead of inviting people to bring a dish, ask them to bring a story, a joke, or a game that will make everyone laugh. Be prepared to get the ball rolling by having some material ready in case your guests are slow to get into it. Resources for humorous material are abundant (see Chapter 13: The Power of Humor).

- If you are invited to dinner, tell the hosts that you would like to bring a dish. Assure them that they should serve whatever they desire along with what you bring. Tell them you would like to bring a dessert, too. Emphasize that it is intended to complement whatever they planned to serve. In this way, you avoid the possibility of being a guest for dinner and having to eat what you don't want or picking at what is served and feeling bad about it. If you know the host or hostess well, consider reminding him or her of what you do not eat. Several of my friends know I have coronary heart disease and that I do not eat foods that are fried, creamy, or highly salted.

- Wear a medical identification bracelet. When your blood glucose gets too low, you may be too disoriented to take care of yourself. The ID bracelet will inform others of what is happening. Shakiness and incoherence are common symptoms of hypoglycemia; the uninformed observer might mistakenly assume you are inebriated and turn away.

- If you have a cell phone, enter the number of the person to be contacted in an emergency in the "contact" list of your phone. Name the entry "ICE," which stands for "In Case of Emergency." Paramedics will automatically look for this entry in your phone if you are unable to give them the information. Also, smart phones have apps designed to help paramedics in an emergency. Vital data—health history, medications, primary person to contact—is entered for paramedics to access in case of a medical crisis.

- Educate someone at your workplace about hypoglycemia. Then, if it occurs, your coworker will understand and act on your behalf.

- Always have something on your person to elevate your blood glucose level if needed. You may start to feel low, but decide that because you are only 20 minutes from home, you will check the level when you get there. Don't assume that nothing will get in your way to create a crisis. Glucose tablets or a handful of hard candy do not take up a lot of room. Always carry something with you to use without hesitation.

- If forgetting is a problem, set the alarm clock function on your mobile device as a reminder. Also, the alarm app can be set to ring throughout the day as a reminder to check your present level of mindfulness. It is easy to drift into a mindless state that can go on for a long time. Hearing the alarm will signal you to be mindful of what you are thinking and doing and will get you to shift from a negative to a positive state of mind if necessary.

- If you tend to eat too much when eating out, ask your server to put half of your meal in a doggie bag before bringing the rest to you. Or tell the server not to serve bread or dessert or whatever your particular weakness might be (French fries or chips). If necessary, you can even tell the server beforehand not to accept any request by you for bread or dessert, no matter how much you insist on it. (However, if you are dining with others, try to make certain that your companions are not denied bread or dessert.)
- Consider ordering first so you are not tempted by what others order.
- If someone's comment triggers anger or another negative feeling, consider reframing your reaction. For example, if you think you have been criticized for not taking appropriate care of your diabetes, the reframe might be, "The person meant well, but he or she obviously doesn't know much about diabetes or me, so I just have to pass it off as another challenge that comes with this condition."

For many individuals, it is difficult to resist overeating when a lot of food is available. Portion control is an effective way to deal with this vulnerability. Do not prepare any more food than you want to eat. If it is practical to cook larger amounts, divide what you prepare into reasonable portions and freeze the individual servings for future meals. For many, portion control is central to diabetes management.

I confess that I tend to eat low-fat frozen yogurt right out of the box. When I do, I always eat too much and feel badly for doing it. When I put a reasonable portion in a dish and return the carton to the freezer, I have taken control and eliminated both the temptation to overindulge and the likelihood of self-imposed stress.

4. *Write a list of strengths.* Become mindful of what you do well. Identify your strengths, and write them on a card to carry with you. When you are faced with a potential stressor, refer to your strengths list. If you're in a tough spot, you will want to deal with it from your best hand, so be prepared. Knowing your strengths reinforces the power you have for dealing with the challenges of diabetes and life in general. Refer to the guidelines below for developing your strengths list.

Skills are a strength (writing, using a computer, negotiating, communicating, and problem solving) as are one's personal traits (flexibility, discipline, determination, patience, and versatility). Other strengths, perhaps less obvious, are enthusiasm, creativity, persistence, and honesty.

When you anticipate the possibility of being caught in an undesirable situation, you can take a proactive position. In doing so, a potential stressor is eliminated. The process is basic: being aware of your vulnerabilities presents the opportunity to choose another path. Making the choice is exercising your power, and with this power, you are taking control of what happens to you.

DEVELOPING MY STRENGTHS LIST

Thoughtfully write answers to each of the following *mindful questions*:

MQ | *What am I good at doing?*

What has worked for me in tough times before?

What works to calm me down when I am upset?

Where can I go that has a comforting, peaceful effect on me?

*Which family members and friends can
I call on for support?*

*Which members of my medical team can
I call on for support?*

*When I have been able to help others,
what strengths have I drawn on?*

Transfer your list of strengths to a small card and carry it with you. Use the list, too, as an incentive to build on, or add to, your range of personal strengths.

CHAPTER 13

The Power of Humor

I f you asked 10 people to give their definition of humor, you might get 10 different answers. Here is a practical definition: humor is an experience that results in laughter, smiling, or a feeling of amusement, along with one or more of the following: a decline in tension, mood elevation, pleasant diversion, or a sense of well-being. So you don't have to laugh to experience humor; you simply have to feel good, with a touch of amusement.

The experience of humor is cognitive, physical, and emotional. It affects the way you think, feel, and act. The use of humor is one of only a few positive defense mechanisms. Everyone has methods for defending themselves from undesirable circumstances. Most defense mechanisms are designed to avoid dealing with what is happening by stifling a feeling or by manipulating thoughts. These methods generally do not work well in the long run. For example, denial is a defense mechanism that attempts to protect us from something that would be too disturbing to bear, as if not facing it will make it go away. In general, however, humor is a safe and comforting way to deal with many difficult situations. It provides an effective alternative to a stress-provoking response. A humorous response is a way of defending oneself from unnecessary anguish without unpleasant consequences.

Is Humor the Best Medicine?

The answer is yes and no. There are times when humor is the best cure for an "ill" situation. There are injuries and illnesses for which humor lightens the burden and, sometimes, even nurtures healing. As an effective stress-buster, mirth and laughter help prevent the onset of some medical conditions. However, for an illness, injury, or disease—physical or mental—humor is not an adequate alternative to medical treatment and medication.

Humor can enrich your health and well-being in numerous ways. A sense of amusement often, but not always, accompanied by laughter, has a direct or indirect effect on your ability to control stress and, thereby, to manage your diabetes. Like most things in life, there is the other side of the coin: humor can have unfavorable consequences when it is used inappropriately. One purpose of this chapter is to help you bring more humor into your life, to make a "sense of humor" a mindful part of your everyday experience, and to make certain that you do not use it in a harmful way. Best of all, mirth and laughter are always a possibility, and they are free.

Using humor to deny the seriousness of a situation would be a poor, if not dangerous, use of mirth and laughter. Think of the person who denies the seriousness of his diabetes with the supposedly lighthearted, carefree attitude: "Hey, something is going to kill you sooner or later, why not diabetes . . . haha." This individual is masking his fearful feelings about diabetes with a desperate joke that could have grim consequences.

Humor is a powerful antidote to stress. The physical and emotional reactions to laughter are counter to the stress response. The experience of amusement elicits a relaxed response, a feeling of well-being, as opposed to the tension and uneasiness common to stress. Certainly, some people find it easier to see the humor in a situation or to make a situation funny. Perhaps you are one of those people who are quick to declare that you just don't have a good sense of humor. It may be true, but it does not mean that you cannot develop the ability to see and appreciate the humorous side of a situation or to be creative and make something funny. Often, the lack of a sense of humor is a result of early conditioning, of receiving messages that create beliefs that oppose the use or appreciation of a fun-loving perspective. In this chapter, you will learn how to overcome the barriers to having a good sense of humor. You will learn how to use fun and laughter both to reduce stress—the nemesis of good diabetes care—and to enrich the quality of your life.

Bottom line, there are circumstances for which humor is not the best medicine; there are few situations for which mirth and laughter are not good for you.

Humor and Living Mindfully

The essence of mindfulness is being awake to where you are, what you are doing, and why you are doing it and knowing if you have a better choice. In this state of mind, you avoid the risks of absentmindedness and of thinking and acting on auto-pilot. Living mindfully is taking the most control of your life possible; mindlessness is giving up control to faulty beliefs, to chance, and to the interests and biases of others.

A mindful person who is in a bad mood or in an undesirable situation does not simply resign herself to what is happening and suffer through it. Being aware both of her undesirable state and the benefits of mirth and laughter, she creates a humorous thought or image to counter the unpleasant mood or situation.

How Can Humor Be Beneficial?

Humor can be a powerful tool for coping with a difficult situation. It reduces and often prevents the stress response. The feeling of amusement accompanied by a smile or laughter has many positive effects on the mind and body, effects that reduce, if not reverse, the intensity of negative emotions. When we see, find, or create a humorous perspective in a difficult situation, we take charge rather than giving in helplessly to what is happening. Humor can enable the control of emotions and feelings that otherwise might spin painfully downward.

Humor can make bearable what otherwise might be unbearable. What do we do when we have lost a loved one? Typically, the eulogy includes humorous stories about the deceased; and we gather in a house of mourning to cry and to recall all the memories of the deceased that make us laugh. It helps us endure the worst of times. You learned in Chapters 1 and 2 how the saber-toothed tigers of modern times—illness, crime, the economy, the well-being of our children or parents, the loss of a loved one—trigger a multitude of unwanted physical and mental changes. Humor can make the tiger toothless and clawless.

The idea that humor is, at the very least, good medicine is not new. Here are several quotes that date back centuries ago and declare the value of mirth and laughter for good health:

> *"To everything there is a season, and a time to every purpose under the heaven: a time to weep, and a time to laugh; a time to mourn, and a time to dance."*

Ecclesiastes 3:4

> *"A merry heart doeth good like a medicine: but a broken spirit drieth the bones."*

Proverbs 17:22

Henri de Mondeville, *a medieval professor of surgery, who lived in the 13th century, wrote, "Let the surgeon take care to regulate the whole regimen of the patient's life for joy and happiness," and he recommended "allowing [patient's] relatives and special friends to cheer him . . . by having someone tell him jokes." He said, too, "The surgeon must forbid anger, hatred, and sadness in the patient."*

Robert Burton, *an English parson and scholar (1577–1640), wrote* Anatomy of Melancholy, *one of the earliest textbooks* of psychiatry. He wrote, "Mirth purges the blood, confirms health, causeth a fresh, pleasing, and fine colour, whets the wit, makes the body young, lively, and fit for any manner of employment."

Immanuel Kant, *the 18th century German philosopher, wrote, "In the case of jokes, we feel the effect of this slackening in the body by the oscillation of the organs, which promotes the restoration of equilibrium and has a favorable influence upon health." Voltaire said that heaven had given us two things to counterbalance the many miseries of life: hope and sleep. Kant said, "He could have added laughter."*

James J. Walsh, *an American physician, published* Laughter and Health *(12), in which he wrote, "The best formula for the health of the individual is contained in the mathematical expression: health varies as the amount of laughter." He wrote, too, "The mental effect brushes away the dreads and fears which constitute the basis of so many diseases or complaints and lifts men out of the slough of despond into which they are so likely to fall when they take themselves overseriously."*

Mark Twain *wrote, "Humor is the great thing, the saving thing, after all. The minute it crops up, all our hardnesses yield, all our irritations and resentments slip away, and the sunny spirit takes their place."*

It has been recognized over the ages that the experience of humor can have important physical, mental, and social benefits. Furthermore, it can be a powerful stabilizer in a crisis.

PHYSICAL BENEFITS OF HUMOR

That feeling of amusement, of lightheartedness, is the opposite of the stress response. Here are some of the positive effects that humor and laughter have on the body:

- Mirth and laughter counteract stress, sparing various bodily systems—including the immune system, the digestive tract, and the coronary system—unnecessary wear and tear.

- Humor enhances healing by activating bodily systems that heal and deactivating systems that oppose healing. It puts body and mind in the right mode for healing.
- A feeling of amusement and laughter decreases pain in three ways:
  - By reducing muscular tension
  - By causing the release of endorphins, the opiate-like polypeptides that are the body's natural painkillers
  - By distracting from the pain
- With laughter, blood pressure rises initially; then it is likely to fall below where it was before laughing.
- Research indicates that humor may help prevent heart disease and heart attacks.
- Laughing increases heart rate, improving circulation. In a study done at the University of Maryland School of Medicine, researchers found that a humorous experience had a positive effect on blood flow, an effect opposite to what occurs with a stressful event. Subjects watched a violent scene from a war movie and a humorous scene from a comedy. The researchers tested the subjects' vasodilation—the ability of the blood vessels to expand—as they watched the two scenes. While watching the battle scene, 14 of 20 subjects had a significant decrease in blood flow, whereas 19 of 20 had a significant increase in blood flow watching the comedy segment. Overall, blood flow dropped by approximately 35% with the stressful war movie. Blood flow increased 22% with the humorous film, which is equivalent to what occurs with a 15- to 30-minute workout. The researchers concluded that there may be a time when it is recognized that a regular 15- to 20-minute period of humor and laughter is as healthy as regular exercise.
- Mirth and laughter foster instant relaxation of mind and body.
- Laughter causes a loss of muscle tone and a release of muscular tension.

- Laughing causes extensive musculoskeletal activity. A hearty laugh exercises the insides.
- Laughter stimulates the digestive tract.
- Mirth and laughter enhance immune function in several ways:
  ○ Decrease cortisol (stress hormone) levels
  ○ Increase levels of infection-fighting immunoglobulin A
  ○ Increase activity of natural killer cells, which seek out and destroy abnormal cells
  ○ More than double levels of plasma cytokine γ-interferon, a protein that enhances immune system function
- As a reliable stress-buster, humor helps a person cope with diabetes more easily and effectively.

MENTAL BENEFITS OF HUMOR

As you learned in Chapter 2, stress has a harmful effect on the mind. In contrast, the positive results produced by a humorous experience soothe and nourish the mind in many ways. Here are some of the ways that mirth and laughter have a positive impact on your mental state.

- Considered to be one of only a few mature defense mechanisms, humor makes facing difficult situations more tolerable. Viewing an unpleasant situation from a humorous perspective gives it a different meaning, one that is less disturbing and more manageable.
- Mirth and laughter are effective antidotes to anger and other distressing emotions. The experience of humor reverses feelings of anger, fear, and shame. These intense feelings cannot share the same mental space with humor at the same time.

A woman who attended my class at the Johns Hopkins Comprehensive Diabetes Center with her husband came back the next day with this story. The previous evening, they had had an argument, and he left the house in a huff. While he was away, she cut a large square hole in a page of the newspaper. When he returned, she met him at the door and put the paper in front of his face saying, "Dr. Napora told us to reframe." They laughed, and the rest of the evening was quite pleasant.

- A sense of humor counters feelings of sadness and reduces the risk of getting depressed. It is a natural mood elevator.
- For those who suffer from taking everything too seriously, laughter quiets the ego and eases the way to inner peace.
- For those who suffer from the need for perfection, humor is a powerful way of letting go and enjoying imperfection. It is the lubricant that eases the friction between the perfection we seek and the reality of who we are with all of our imperfections.
- A sense of humor helps us accept all of our vulnerabilities, to turn away from pretentiousness and pomposity. In a state of mirth, we can see our fragility from a safe place and, thus, accept it.

Carrie Grady, the Johns Hopkins University freshman who was quoted in Chapter 7, told me how her friends use humor to help her deal with diabetes. When she is showing signs of hypoglycemia, they will playfully say something like, "Uh oh, Carrie is going low on us," which creates a shared amusement that is much more constructive than if they simply insist that her blood glucose level is low and she has to do something about it. She added that their teasing approach works because she knows that they take diabetes very seriously.

- Humor allows one to channel adversity into something positive. It is not uncommon for people with serious handicaps to make a joke about their affliction. Being able to laugh at oneself counters the possibility of making something so serious that it becomes overwhelmingly distressing.
- A mirthful perspective makes fearful situations more manageable. Soldiers in combat, prisoners of war, and

hostages have used humor to comfort themselves in very tough times. Hospital nurses are known to poke fun among themselves at their ill patients—not out of disrespect or a lack of sensitivity, but rather to get relief from observing horrendous sickness that someday could be their fate.

- The process of finding or creating the humor in a situation fosters creative thinking in other areas of functioning. Creativity involves seeing a possibility other than what is apparent, which is similar to finding the humor in a situation that would not otherwise have been amusing.
- Humor can provide relief from suffering the loss of a loved one.
- Laughing feels good and is contagious. Later in this chapter, you will be encouraged to participate in a laughter club, which is a group of people who meet simply to laugh together. The stimulus of consistently hearty laughter spreads rapidly.
- A humorous state reduces the risk of behaving inappropriately, which is a risk when someone is feeling resentful, frightened, or ashamed.

Each of these mental benefits directly or indirectly reduces stress, which enhances your ability to maintain healthy glucose levels.

In *Anatomy of an Illness* (13), Norman Cousins tells of recovering from an extremely painful disease that was considered by experts to be irreversible. He attributed his recovery, in large part, to occupying himself with humorous material. Cousins wrote, "It makes little sense to suppose that emotions exact only penalties and confer no benefits . . . the positive emotions are life-giving experiences."

To earn the degree of Doctor of Philosophy, I was required to conduct original research. I chose to write my thesis, *A Study of the Effects of a Program of Humorous Activity on the Subjective Well-Being of Senior Adults* (14). Two groups of senior citizens attended a six-week program, with the experimental group participating in humorous activities and the control group taking part in discussions on various topics. Because of the limits of this short-term study, the data did not provide any conclusions about possible long-term benefits of a humorous experience. However, the data over the course of the project indicated that levels of mood and other measures of personal satisfaction increased significantly after each session and over the course of the study. These positive results occurred for both groups but significantly more so for the humor group. Although not considered scientific evidence of the benefits of humor, I can report that participants in the humor group did not want me to stop the program.

SOCIAL BENEFITS OF HUMOR

Any of the benefits of humor listed thus far can pave the way for positive social interactions. However, mirth and laughter can have such a powerful influence on social relations that they require separate consideration. Here are some of the ways that humor can enrich your social experiences.

- Humor is a great "icebreaker." As the renowned comedian Victor Borge said, "Laughter is the shortest distance between two people." When two or more individuals laugh at the same thing, they experience a commonality. They feel a connection; differences are minimized. Public speakers, for example, almost always start a presentation with a joke because it quickly establishes a pleasant rapport with an audience.
- Because humor reduces tension and stress, it is an effective tool for ending disagreements without undue strife. Families, friends, coworkers, and any group that has a common cause need humor in their repertoire.

  This is a great example told in Psyching Out Diabetes: A Positive Approach to Your Negative Emotions (15), coauthored by my dear friend and colleague Dr. Richard Rubin (may he rest in peace), whose son Stefan has type 1 diabetes. Stefan was diagnosed at age 9 and did remarkably well coping with diabetes until he had to take a shot of insulin at dinnertime. He was not happy about the second injection and made it clear, protesting vigorously every evening before dinner. His father did everything he could think of to convince Stefan of the reason it was necessary and in his best interest. The drama went on for weeks. One evening, Stefan asked again, "Why can't I just take one shot a day?" Frustrated and annoyed, Dr. Rubin was about to try once more to respond with some convincing data; instead, he asked if Stefan would prefer to take the insulin just once a week. His son was intrigued and countered, "How about one shot a month?" Finally agreeing to one shot a year, Stefan calculated that the dose of insulin would be 12,775 units. They laughed heartily, Stefan took his shot without complaining, and he never protested again.

- It has been said that "people who pray together, stay together." It is equally true that "people who play together, stay together." Many couples have told me that it was their shared sense of humor that got them through some very difficult times. In fact, many individuals who were asked what they wanted most in a spouse answered, "a sense of humor."

- Humor makes imperfection acceptable. The perception of imperfections is a common source of strife in relationships, but when the expectation of perfection is seen for its absurdity, it becomes harmless and laughable. Sometimes, the realization of imperfection in oneself or another is even a source of bonding.

There was a story on television about a young girl who was being treated for cancer. Because of chemotherapy, she was totally bald, which might have been very embarrassing for this young person, except that her family and many of her classmates shaved their heads. Their laughter put the situation into perspective. Their act created a sense of solidarity and mocked any pretense of self-importance.

- Because laughter is contagious, it can unite a family or any gathering of people. Joviality is common in support groups. Individuals who tend to be anxious in social situations are likely to find relief in a group that is jolly as opposed to being in a tense, overly serious environment.

HUMOR AND CRISIS

Among the most amazing and inspiring examples of human strength and resilience are the stories of those who have endured incredible hardships and who have used humor as an essential means of survival. Many prisoners of war, hostages, and the physically challenged—those who have been thrust into emotional crises—have attributed their survival, in part, to being able to find or create a humorous perspective in otherwise unbearable circumstances.

Remember when Republican President Ronald Reagan was shot in an attempted assassination? Going into surgery, he said that he hoped the surgeon was not a Democrat. Not knowing if he would survive the injury, he made a joke of his predicament—hopefully creating a brief diversion from the crisis.

Condemned to a Nazi concentration camp, Viktor Frankl in *Man's Search for Meaning* (6) wrote, "Humor was another of the soul's weapons in the fight for self-preservation. It is well known that humor, more than anything else in the human make-up, can afford an aloofness and an ability to rise above any situation, even if only for a few seconds."

In Chapter 9: The Frame of Letting Go, you were introduced to Arnold Beiser, who had graduated from medical school at the age of 23 and had won a national tennis championship a year later. Shortly afterward, he contracted polio and became quadriplegic—unable to walk or to practice medicine. His ability to overcome a series of incredible hardships is a remarkable story of courage, determination, and self-examination. In *Flying Without Wings* (7), in an account of his ordeal, Beiser emphasizes the role of humor in dealing with his condition. He wrote, "I still feel relief, and my sense of well-being is restored whenever I laugh or find something to smile about. It gives me a new perspective on life; what an instant before seemed insurmountable and tragic becomes quite acceptable." Beiser also wrote, "Humor is a great equalizer, elevating the victim to the level of the perpetrator, diminishing the self-inflated, and showing the kinship among people. It also shows that tragedy and comedy are but two aspects of what is real, and whether we see the tragic or the humorous is a matter of perspective."

One of the most common emotional crises, one that everyone experiences, is the loss of a loved one. It is generally a time of agonizing psychological pain and heart-wrenching grief. It is also a time that evokes memories of the deceased, both sad and humorous. Eulogies, intended to pay tribute, are likely to contain recollections that stimulate laughter. Family and friends join together and tearfully recount memories of the deceased that provoke laughter and relief.

Each of the benefits of humor listed above can help an individual cope with a crisis, even if only for moments at a time. The distraction, a shift in perspective, and the ability to laugh at one's predicament takes us away from feelings of fear and despair, as Frankl said, "even if only for a few seconds."

NEGATIVE EFFECTS OF HUMOR

There are circumstances in which the use of humor is not appropriate, when mirth and laughter can be harmful.

- Humor should not be used to deny the seriousness of a situation. Joking about poor self-control—"Well, you have to die from something"—is not only irrational, it is also dangerous. Having diabetes is serious and requires thoughtful attention. Humor can ease the burden of dealing with diabetes, but managing the disease has to be dealt with . . . period.
- Humor should be used thoughtfully. Know your audience. Use humor that everyone present can enjoy. The physically challenged often make fun of their

afflictions, but someone with a handicap may not appreciate a joke about their condition when it is made by someone who does not have the same disability.

- Humor can, and often is, used to express hostility. Be alert to humor that pokes fun at or puts down anyone, a group, or a cause. Be mindful of jokes that negatively portray a religion, ethnicity, or nationality. Are they meant to be harmful or are they an attempt to mask the joker's hostility? Hopefully, telling a hostile joke or laughing at one would lead you to ask yourself, "What is going on, and do I want to be a part of it?"

- When humor is used indirectly to convey a message, the intended message may be missed or misunderstood by the recipient. Your annoyance may not come across by telling your critic that you are going to have to call friends in Chicago if he doesn't stop telling you what you shouldn't eat. He may not get the joke that "friends in Chicago" refers to the mafia and that they would make sure he stopped criticizing you. It is a risk to assume that someone will get the message; it is more likely to be understood when the message is direct: "If you don't stop criticizing what I eat, I'm not going to want to be with you."

- Laughing at oneself is positive when you do it as a reminder to not take yourself too seriously. It is unhealthy when you use it to degrade yourself or to deny you made a mistake.

- From childhood we learn that being amusing can ingratiate us with others, especially with peers. Getting a laugh from others by poking fun at someone can be very tempting, but it is cruel and weak behavior. A healthy use of humor is a sure way to win friends and influence people.

- People in deep depression or who suffer from mania or other mental disorders are not likely to respond favorably to an attempt at humor.

- There are some physical conditions for which hearty laughter can be undesirable. Individuals with breathing problems—asthma or bronchitis—or who have had recent surgery or other conditions such as spinal disc disease, urinary incontinence, and hernias can have unpleasant reactions from laughing too strongly.

Humor in Action

Using humor to manage the stress of diabetes does not require becoming a good joke-teller or having to find humor in everything that happens. Diabetes can be tough on the nerves, and laughing it off is not always an option. But having a humorous perspective will help minimize stress, easing life's trials and tribulations. Mirth and laughter often can be an adaptive approach to hardship. Having a comic view of life's ups and downs—without denying the seriousness of the situation—reduces the risk of overreacting to the many challenges of diabetes and life.

Psychologist Sheila Krystal said, "You are only one thought away from a good feeling." Making that thought a funny one is always a choice. You do not have to be born with a sense of humor. Commit to making humor an important part of your daily life and you may be surprised at how much fun you can have.

A woman told the following story at a diabetes workshop. Her father has diabetes, and over time, diabetes had seriously damaged his kidneys. He had taken a test that would determine whether he had to go on dialysis. She was terrified at the prospect of her father needing that treatment, anticipating that he would be devastated if he had to do it. They met with the doctor, who informed them that he indeed needed dialysis. She felt a wave of horror, which quickly subsided when her father said, "That's alright doc; I have three daughters, and I never could get the bathroom when I needed it." Then, she felt a strong wave of relief, certain that her father would be able to deal with the treatments.

Seeing the humor in a situation is always a possibility. It is an alternative that saves us from the futility of one-possibility reactions to difficult situations. Make a commitment to developing a mirthful spirit. Practice finding and creating a humorous perspective, especially in situations that can cause you distress. Be mindful of your feelings, and when they are discomforting, be *mindful* that a humorous frame can reduce, and perhaps relieve, the uneasiness.

Eating is the primary social event in most cultures. Getting together for dinner, for a picnic, or for happy hour are typical social events that challenge the individual with diabetes. How about "bring a funny story" rather than "bring a dish" as the theme of a gathering? This will make laughter, not food, the focus of the evening. When food is the only attraction, it is human nature to get carried away and make it an excessive indulgence.

Make mirth and laughter integral parts of each day. Mindfully find and create humor until it becomes as natural as brushing your teeth. Have fun with it. You do not have to be born with a sense of humor to make it work for you now.

How Can I Develop a Sense of Humor?

I believe that everyone has the right stuff for developing a healthy sense of humor. However, for some, there are barriers to being mirthful. Messages received in childhood, such as "grow up" and "stop acting like a child," can become beliefs that forbid being mirthful: "It is dangerous for me to laugh and be playful" or "If I want approval, then I have to be serious about everything." As you are learning from this book, these types of frames can be very forceful even though they are senseless.

Start developing a sense of humor with these *mindful questions*:

MQ | *How much was humor and laughter encouraged or discouraged when I was growing up?*

*Who has made the biggest
impression on me, and
did he or she have a good
sense of humor?*

*What did I learn in the past
that diminishes my sense
of humor?*

Knowing what the barriers are to having a sense of humor
will prepare you to minimize or, perhaps, avoid such
barriers.

Once you know the barriers, you can take the steps needed
to develop a sense of humor or to enrich the sense of humor
you already have. Whether your objective is to change from
little or no sense of humor to some sense of humor or from a
good sense of humor to a great one, any change begins with
making a commitment to change. Then, you must make mindful choices that lead to the changes you desire.

MQ   *What are my beliefs about
having fun, about laughing,
and about being childlike?*

*If my belief opposes a type of
humor, is my attitude plausible?*

*How can I reframe a senseless
belief to be comfortable and
inviting of mirth and laughter?
(How about, "Not everyone who
has a good sense of humor came
to it naturally. Like other skills,
I have learned by my own effort;
I will develop this one, too.")*

*Are there types of humor—
anecdotal, farcical, satirical,
surreal, improvisational,
topical, dark—that I prefer?*

*Can I make a commitment
to have at least a few mirthful
experiences each day?*

PRACTICE, PRACTICE, PRACTICE

Having made a commitment to developing your sense of humor, the ensuing task—like cultivating any skill—is to practice as much as possible. Here are some ways to make humor a bigger part of each day:

- Start the day by reading the comics in your newspaper. If your paper does not have a comics section or it isn't enough, there are boundless comic sites on the Internet. I use gocomics.com, which has just about every comic strip and single panel gag ever published, and it is free (with advertisements). Google "cartoons," "jokes," or "comics" to find numerous sources of fun and laughter. It may take some sorting out, but these sites have a vast selection of material to enjoy.

- Make finding and creating humor a game. When you're stuck in traffic, waiting endlessly in your doctor's office, or in a line that is moving slower than molasses, look around and find someone who is in the same situation and is about to explode. Imagine that she does . . . oh, what a mess. No harm intended, just lightening up a bit.

- Keep a humor journal. Record funny experiences, stories, and jokes. Try your hand at creating a humorous story, poem, or cartoon. Include family pictures that you have given your personal touch by adding a humorous caption for each photo.

- Visit a bookstore and look at some of the books in the Humor section. See what makes you laugh. See what style of humor tickles you the most. Do you like cartoons, comic strips, topical humor, funny stories, word play, puns, or limericks? Which type of humor is most joyful? When you find your favorites, make them a part of each day, even if only for a few minutes.

- Start a book club that only selects literature that is light-hearted and humorous. You will not run out of good material in your lifetime.
- Start a laughter club. These clubs are centered on regular social gatherings in which the sole purpose is for the participants to bring something to amuse the group. Conclude each meeting with a giggle segment. Have someone start to laugh, even if it is forced. You will be amazed at how it will rapidly reach everyone there. Remember, laughter is contagious.
- If starting a laughter club is not practical, consider joining one of the clubs that already exist around the world. Dr. Madan Kataria created the first laughter club in 1995. Now, there are more than 5,000 clubs around the world. At club meetings, members just start laughing—not at a joke or cartoon, but simply for the sake of laughing. The clubs operate on a simple principle: laughter begets laughter. "Yoga laughter" groups have grown out of the original laughter clubs. In these gatherings, unconditional laughter is combined with yogic breathing. Laughter is simulated as a body exercise in a group using eye contact and childlike playfulness that quickly turns into real laughter. Their practice is supported by scientific data that have shown that the physiological and psychological benefits are the same for real and pretend laughter. Information about laughter and yoga laughter groups can be found on the Internet.
- Do something outrageously silly when you are annoyed or in a bad mood. Dance like a whirling dervish or pretend you are a cheerleader, cheering for yourself, of course.
- Remind yourself to keep things in perspective. When you feel bad about something, consider how you have

exaggerated some aspect of the situation, and then exaggerate it even more. For example, suppose you were at a diabetes support group, and you made a comment that was not well received. It made you feel bad. It is likely that you are exaggerating the reaction of the other group members, perhaps thinking that they think you are stupid. With this in mind, exaggerate the idea even more by imagining that after the meeting they are calling each other to say how dumb you are and that it will even be a headline in the newspaper tomorrow and certainly everywhere on the Internet. This is an example of taking oneself too seriously, and by exaggerating your thinking even more, you can laugh at yourself for getting caught up in it. The reality is that the other group members are not thinking about you at all . . . darn it.

- Create a mantra—a statement that affirms your self-worth in a humorous way—and recite it often. How about these? "I may not be perfect, but some of my parts are beautiful," or, "Once, I wished I was someone else, and oh what a mess." Another favorite is, "I'm not OK, you're not OK, and that's OK."

- Play a game. Here is one that only takes minutes to set up. Select some cartoons from the newspaper or magazines, and make enough copies without the captions for the number of people who will play. Number the cartoons, so that all the ones that are the same have the same number. Give each player a set of the cartoons and paper and pencil. Have each player write a caption for each cartoon and sign them. One person, acting as facilitator, gathers the sets of cartoons. Then, the leader reads the captions for each cartoon without identifying the authors. The players are asked to guess who wrote each caption. The one who gets the most right is the winner. The fun peaks with a discussion of why specific captions were attributed to specific individuals. Imagine that someone has written a somewhat risqué caption that several other players attribute to the wrong person.

- Recall an embarrassing experience, and write it down. Discover or create a humorous perspective for what happened. Use exaggeration and drama freely to make the rewrite of your experience as funny as possible.

TRACK, EVALUATE, AND ENJOY

In the pursuit of any goal, it is important to evaluate your progress. Here is a way to evaluate the effectiveness of your effort. Keep score with this system:

ACTIVITY	POINTS
Smile	1
Laugh	3
Tell a joke	4
Play a fun game with someone	8
Watch a comedy movie or a television sitcom; read a humorous book	10
Go to a comedy club or your own humor group	30

How are you doing? Is your score higher today than it was yesterday? Is it better this week than last week? If not, what do you need to do to raise your score?

If you are stuck trying to find or create a humorous perspective, try these *mindful questions*:

MQ | *Am I still a victim of faulty beliefs that keep me from enjoying humor?*

What belief or beliefs do I need to reframe?

Do I need to review this chapter to see if I missed something that would help me to get unstuck?

A friend and colleague would periodically remind me and others that "blessings abound." Indeed they do, and humor and laughter are a blessing for everyone to enjoy. They are everywhere to be harvested and consumed. Make it a passion in your life. In Chapter 7: Choosing the Style in Lifestyle, you were encouraged to make your lifestyle a mindful choice and to have a purpose or purposes for everything you do. Make humor and laughter a purpose every day; they are magical stress-busters.

The value of humor is captured most heartily and humorously with this quote from A.L. Rautman, a mental health specialist:

A sense of humor is like the spring under a lumber wagon: It does not lighten the load. It does not make the grating sound of the wheels on the gravel less noisy or harsh. It does not make less of a strain on the horse's neck. But the wagon spring does make the entire ride easier on your rear end.

CHAPTER 14

The Internet: Excellent with Caution

You either use the Internet or you are backward.

~Lee Kuan Yew

I would add a few words to Mr. Yew's take on the Internet: "Maybe, yes, maybe not . . . depends on how you use it." Used wisely, the Internet is a phenomenal source of information and an incredible means of communication. Unfortunately, the Internet is also an uncontrollable system for misinformation and for brutally hateful assaults from anonymous evildoers. The Internet offers access to numerous diabetes-related resources that can aid in managing diabetes. Websites and alternative online sources (portals, podcasts and apps) offer sound information and advice; however, users must make certain that the website is an authentic and reliable source.

What Is the Internet?

The Internet is a configuration of networks that connect millions of computers together globally. It creates a system in which any electronic device can communicate with another as long as they are connected to the Internet. The World Wide Web (WWW), or the Web, is a way of accessing information over the Internet. (Other ways to access information include email and instant messaging.)

A search engine is a software system designed to help users find websites and other information on the Web. There are numerous search engines including Google, Bing, and DuckDuckGo. Browsers retrieve and display web pages, images, and videos on a user's device. Popular browsers include Firefox, Safari, Internet Explorer, Opera, and Google Chrome; these browsers are generally formatted to a specific operating system, such as Microsoft Windows, Apple iOS, and Google's Android OS.

The Need for Empowerment

Although you may have the services of a well-rounded team of professional care providers, managing diabetes is fundamentally your responsibility. The task—or perhaps more succinctly, the demand—for someone with diabetes is to keep blood glucose levels within a healthy range at least most of the time. This endeavor is replete with obstacles: a lack of pertinent knowledge, an incompatible disposition, an unhealthy lifestyle, an inordinate amount of stress, poor access to essential services, and the costs of medicines, supplies, devices, and services. The consequences for poor self-management can be grim, if not tragic.

Fortunately, there has been a continuous effort by hospitals, medical associations, scientists, pharmaceutical companies, device manufacturers, and technology enterprises to help people with diabetes achieve successful management of their malady. Their mission is to empower the patient by enhancing individual competence and autonomy. Internet technology is focused, too, on lowering the cost of patient care and easing the burden on providers related to the time required to answer inquiries.

The Role of the Internet in Diabetes Self-Management

The Internet can provide information, support, feedback, and, in some cases, direct assistance to people with diabetes. Online programs provide self-assessment tools and ways to monitor factors central to good glucose management. These factors include blood glucose level, insulin dosage, physical activity, weight, and state of mind. Diabetes orientation support groups are available that provide an opportunity to discuss problems and solutions with others. Internet and Web-based programs complement traditional physician-centered care; they provide options that are more fluid, real-time, and patient-focused services. Online services can provide feedback and guidance to patients between in-person visits. However, the developers of these programs continue to resolve inherent problems for both patients and providers. Despite current and potential benefits of Internet-based self-management services, some of the systems and strategies currently available require caution, which will be described throughout this chapter.

Professional care providers, too, are empowered by advances in technology that enable more frequent evaluation of data sent to them about the patient's performance and physical status. With the range of resources and accessibility of the Internet, clinicians have the means to greatly improve a patient's ability to effectively self-manage his or her diabetes. Like any momentous and fast-developing phenomenon, there are still problems affecting providers that need to be resolved, such as time spent and costs for their services.

APPS

An app (application) is a computer program that is downloaded to mobile devices. There are more than 1,100 iOS and Android diabetes-oriented apps available on the Apple App Store and Google Play. Apps provide a variety of services to assist someone with diabetes in achieving and maintaining good glycemic levels. Specifically, these programs have various goals:

- To educate the patient about the disease and how to manage it.
- To provide real-time glucose readings, trends, and alerts regarding undesired glucose levels.

- To facilitate communication with a doctor or other care providers to get quick, if not real-time, assistance.
- To transmit data—glycemic results, intake of insulin and other medications, actual time of entries, and other relevant information—to a clinician or service organization.
- To receive feedback and advice based on the data sent to a professional care provider.
- To provide information about eating healthfully, nutritional data, and countless recipes attuned to glycemic management.
- To provide guidance, motivation, and performance data regarding physical activity.
- To receive periodic messages intended to motivate and inspire parents to maintain a regimen consistent with healthy glycemic management.
- To access a diabetes-oriented support group.

Many apps are free, at least for the startup version. However, a fee is not uncommon for advanced renditions of a program. Frequently, the extra charge is simply to eliminate commercial advertisements.

For Apple and Android users alike, if you are not certain about how to perform a task, open your search engine—Google, Safari, Bing, etc.—and type in the question you want answered. For example, "How to search for an app?" Keep it simple: "How to select and get an app?" rather than "What do I have to do to select and download an app of my choice?" Most apps are a component of an enterprise that uses a website as its base.

WEBSITES

Specific websites are highly recommended for two reasons: 1) they offer a vast amount of information and services and 2) they are unquestionably reliable. Each of the following websites is a product of a highly recognized health and diabetes organization:
- diabetes.org (American Diabetes Association)
- niddk.nih.gov (National Institute of Diabetes and Digestive and Kidney Diseases—NIDDK)

- joslin.org (Joslin Diabetes Center)
- diabeteseducator.org (American Association of Diabetes Educators—AADE)
- https://medlineplus.gov (National Library of Medicine— National Institutes of Health)
- healthfinder.gov (Office of Disease Prevention and Health Promotion in the U.S. Department of Health and Human Services)

In addition to the prominent websites listed above, there are other organizations that deserve mention:

- healthline.com is a destination site for health and wellness information over a wide range of subjects and services.
- webmd.com also offers information for a variety of medical issues. In addition to its website, WebMD offers an app that can be downloaded to a mobile device for ready access.
- onedrop.today features a number of services including an app that can be linked to any of your devices. The app offers assistance with medication scheduling, meal planning, exercising, and "automated decision support" among other things.
- dexcom.com offers a glucose monitoring system that provides real-time data that allows you to proactively manage your diabetes.

Unless your doctor or clinic recommends a specific monitoring system, take the time to explore some of these sites. Most of the websites and corresponding apps are very similar, but there may be a feature that is especially appealing to you. And there may be fees for certain services. To start looking or to make a final decision, it would be wise to check on the site below:

- danaapps.org, a feature of the American Association of Diabetes Educators, evaluates health-related apps. Tap on a subject such as "diabetes" and the site provides a number of apps that have undergone exhaustive examination. Each app is rated *average, good,* or *excellent.*

> Caution: Any app or website is not a substitute for consulting your medical team if you are experiencing unexplained discomfort.

There usually are multiple links at the bottom of a home page of a website—links that access other sections and services of the organization. There also will be a link that enables you to "Contact Us," which provides the means for communicating via email or phone and, occasionally, to chat directly with a representative of the organization.

PORTALS

A portal is a "personal" website that connects physicians and their patients. The content of a portal is login-protected and user-specific, meaning that the data are accessible only to the user and the providers who sponsor the service. Its purpose is to both promote and empower patients' involvement in managing their diabetes. (Portals are available for many chronic illnesses and other medical conditions.) A typical portal features various disease management tools:

- View most lab results as soon as they are available
- Renew prescriptions
- Exchange secure email messages with care providers
- View summaries of office and/or hospital visits
- View upcoming appointments
- Pay your physician and/or hospital bill

Patients forward records of their blood glucose levels, blood pressure, and body weight to the provider, who monitors these vital health data. The typical portal is an interactive system for exchanging information between patients and providers. Patients may also have a place to organize their personal health records: contact information, medical and family history, medication details, lifestyle choices, and test results. Portals are intended to encourage and facilitate involvement of patients in their diabetes care.

PODCASTS

A podcast is a series of digital audio and video files that are not offered on a fixed schedule. The American Diabetes Association (diabetes.org), for example, produces a podcast of real-life stories of overcoming challenges by people living with type 2 diabetes. National Public Radio (npr.org) offers several podcasts, with some on the topic of diabetes management. You can search "diabetes podcasts" on your browser for other presentations, being cautious about the source of the material. Avoid apps that promise to "reverse" diabetes. The "Podcast App" provides access to most, if not all, available podcasts. The January/February (2019) issue of *Diabetes Forecast* presents a list of podcasts that they consider to be the best concerning diabetes. This list is included in the Resources in Part 5 of this book.

TEXT MESSAGING

Text messaging, or texting, is the act of composing and sending electronic messages, originally consisting of alphabetic and numeric characters, between two or more users of mobile devices, desktops/laptops, or other types of compatible computers. Text messages may be sent over a cellular network, or they may also be sent via the Internet. Texting has grown beyond alphanumeric text to include multimedia messages containing digital images, videos, and sound content, as well as ideograms known as emoji (happy faces, sad faces, and other icons).

Text messaging is an effective means for interacting with others, often in real time. Some medical practices and diabetes clinics are set up to receive and respond to texts from their patients. Also, two or more acquaintances with diabetes can readily communicate via cell phones, exchanging information and offering support to one another. Texting is a well-received means of connecting people with a common interest, regardless of their location.

SUPPORT GROUPS

Living with diabetes is not only physically challenging, it often involves psychological strain and emotional distress. One of the best antidotes for feeling overwhelmed by something is to have the support of others who can understand your agitated state because they have been there. Trust develops quickly knowing that members of the group have a firsthand understanding of your condition. Having the support of others with the same ailment builds strength and a comforting sense of belonging.

Many hospitals and diabetes clinics conduct support groups. For someone who does not have a group available to attend directly, there are online opportunities. Type "diabetes support group" into your search engine or browser and consider what is available.

To decide which diabetes support group is best for you, speak to or text the person running the group, asking these *mindful questions:*

MQ | *What is your background and your qualifications for your role in the group?*

What is the purpose of the group, and how is it run?

Have a list of your specific goals for attending the group. Do your objectives coincide with that of the group?

Reliable websites that offer group activity are:
- https://community.diabetes.org/home (American Diabetes Association)
- joslin.org (Joslin Diabetes Center)
- diabetes.co.uk (National Health Services, United Kingdom)
- https://beyondtype1.org/the-power-of-community/ (Beyond Type 1 support community)

Valid or Not?

The Internet is a vast source of genuine knowledge. But, user beware. Remember that some apps and websites are hoaxes or fraudulent, and therefore potentially dangerous. Content on the Internet is not regulated; anyone can publish whatever they choose. For this reason, some individuals and entities intentionally use this platform to deceive the user, often for personal profit.

When using the Internet for medical information or advice, it is essential to know that the source is authentic. If the publisher is not a renowned institution, a deep-rooted association, a nationally recognized medical center, or a federal agency, be *mindfully* curious. Use these ***mindful questions*** to sort out the good from the bad:

MQ | *Is the publisher a well-recognized health organization or a government agency, or, at the very least, associated with a reliable agency? What does the "About Us" section note concerning the origin, purpose, and resources of the site?* (This section of a website may be at the top of the first page or at the bottom of the last page of the site.)

When was the page published or last updated? (Be cautious of material that may not be current. New, scientifically supported information is ongoing, and it is important that websites present the most recent findings.)

Does the site make health claims that seem too good to be true? (Trust your instincts and seek more information about the source before accepting it as valid.)

Does the site guarantee quick, miraculous results? Does it use a dramatic writing style with certain words emphasized with a bold font, capital letters, or exclamation points? (The information may be presented in a way that plays on the reader's emotions.)

Does the site protect my privacy? (There should be a link saying "Privacy" or "Privacy Policy" that will inform you of any risks to using the site. If the policy includes sharing your information with commercial enterprises, then your personal data is not protected.)

Does the personal information required to "sign in" or "log in" to a site make sense? Why do they need to have my credit card data or social security number?

Is there a bias to this site? Is the site's originator a pharmaceutical company, a diabetes device manufacturer, or business selling a product or services? (If so, this does not necessarily make the site unacceptable; it is, however, a signal to exercise caution.)

Am I uneasy about this website? (If there is any doubt about the validity of material on the site or, simply, a bad gut feeling, try another website or consult your professional care providers.)

The Internet and Stress Management

Stress is poison to diabetes. This message is repeated throughout this book. Coping with the disease is very stressful. Whether it is diabetes-related stress or the psychological strain of family, work, or lifestyle, the results impede the effort to achieve glycemic control. The problem is cyclical: diabetes brings on harmful stress, and stress makes diabetes management more difficult. (See Chapters 1 and 2 for comprehensive information about stress and its impact on managing the disease.)

Health problems caused or exacerbated by stress include:
- Depression and anxiety
- Pain of any kind
- Sleep difficulties
- Autoimmune diseases
- Digestive problems
- Skin conditions, such as eczema
- Heart disease
- Weight issues
- Reproductive issues
- Thinking and memory problems

Any one of these conditions—or a combination thereof, which is highly probable—will discourage, distract from, and defeat the effort to maintain a healthy diabetes regimen. Consistent with the fundamental purpose of *The Mindful Guide to Managing Diabetes*, the Internet offers various apps and websites to help users recognize their distress and implement ways to reduce or eliminate their physical tension and emotional strain. (Internet sources for using meditation to relieve stress are presented in Chapter 15, along with other means of meditating.)

APPS

Approaches to stress management on the Internet include:

- Self-help strategies with or without access to the community for support
- Nature sounds along with enchanting music and/or a mesmerizing visual display for relaxation
- Analysis of sleep patterns to improve rest and alleviate anxiety
- Information and techniques for moderating panic attacks
- A log to record the user's emotions and the triggers that cause stress and anxiety in real time
- Creative activities (e.g., images for adults to color) to alleviate anxiety
- Means to anonymously seek emotional support and counseling from "trained" active listeners
- Games and activities for fun and for letting go of stress and physical tension
- Guided meditation

To evaluate or adopt a stress-oriented app, follow the same routine presented in the section on diabetes-related apps above.

WEBSITES

Numerous websites offer extensive information and advice regarding the interactions of stress and diabetes. It simply is not practical to catalog the collection of sites. An effective way to find the sites that are right for you is to type "stress and diabetes" into your search engine or browser. With patience and perseverance, you will find one or more sites that satisfy your interests. Although the publishers of most of these websites seem to be legitimate, some caution should be exercised when using the Internet. Websites published by well-recognized institutions and professional associations are genuine, safe choices.

These **mindful questions** will help you to stay focused in pursuing information about the connections between stress and diabetes:

MQ | *What specifically am I looking for in surfing these websites?* (Write down your answer and refer to it frequently so you are not drawn off course by the promotions and advertisements that appear on your screen.)

Would it be helpful to review the same subject in this book (check the Index)? (As someone once said, "Two heads are better than one.")

If my needs or concerns have not been satisfied, who might provide clarification?

There is a pressing need to encourage and to empower people with diabetes to play a larger role in managing their blood glucose and the disease in general. It is estimated that more than 500,000,000 people were living with diabetes all over the world in 2018. In 2015, 30.3 million Americans, or 9.4% of the population, had diabetes, and approximately 7.2 million were undiagnosed. About 1.25 million American children and adults had type 1 diabetes. It is estimated that 1.5 million Americans are diagnosed with diabetes every year. In 2015, 84.1 million Americans age 18 and older had prediabetes. The total costs of diagnosed diabetes in the United States in 2017 was estimated to be $327 billion.

Patients with diabetes have increased risks of cardio-vascular disease, renal failure, neurological conditions, and retinopathy. Despite these dire risks and despite the fact that improving glycemic management reduces the risk of complications, a significant number of people with the disease are not managing it well. According to the National Diabetes Statistics Report (2017), a publication of the Centers for Disease Control and Prevention, U.S. Department of Health and Human Services, 15.6% of adults had an A1C value higher than 9%. The American Diabetes Association recommends a level of 7% or less.

This chapter has explored the potential of the Internet to help patients achieve and maintain good diabetes management. Many obstacles to glycemic regulation—lack of information, lack of accessibility, absence of the support of others who share the same problems, and the stressful nature of the disease—are being reduced by access to the World Wide Web, the Internet, and its various renditions. With access to the Internet (89% of the population of developing countries have cell phones and 128% [yes, more than one phone per person] of developed countries have them), patients have at hand services that did not exist a decade ago. The Internet is a valuable resource for achieving better management of stress and diabetes. With more research and advancements in Internet resources, it can only get better.

As a means of acquiring information, as a source of communication and human contact, as a means of getting services that are otherwise inaccessible, the Internet is boundless; and it won't stop growing any time soon, if ever.

CHAPTER 15

Mindful Meditation Plus

Why Meditate?

The practice of meditation began in ancient times and is used extensively in many parts of the world. It has maintained a broad following because of its health benefits, because it is so simple that it can be self-taught, and because it is free. Meditating is a powerful technique for controlling tension and stress and, thus, is an effective means of maintaining good diabetes management. Meditating is effective in making the discomforts of diabetes, such as neuropathic pain, less troublesome. In addition, the practice of meditation disciplines the mind. The practice of meditation is a means for controlling the mind, for choosing and sustaining focus and not letting the mind operate haphazardly. Given the many demands of diabetes, the benefits of meditation are especially important.

Specifically, meditation can be used to:
- Release physical tension
- Reduce and prevent stress
- Induce positive emotions
- Heal physical damage
- Reduce physical pain
- Enhance health
- Lower blood pressure
- Energize the body
- Enhance immune system function
- Improve concentration

- Facilitate sleep
- Blunt sensitivity to stress hormones
- Soothe intense emotions
- Reduce emotional reactivity
- Release anger and moderate road rage
- Increase tolerance of illness
- Improve physical performance
- Minimize fatigue and burnout
- Enhance creativity
- Support personal exploration and growth

It should be noted that although there are studies to support each of these benefits of meditation, overall, the research is scientifically inconclusive. The problem is a lack of well-controlled studies, in large part, because the means and results of meditation can vary so much from person to person.

Many of the benefits listed above have both short-term and long-term rewards. For example, meditating can quickly reduce tension and stress. Thus, practicing the technique over time tends to reduce susceptibility to being tense or unnerved. And the more you practice, the easier it becomes to relax and to reap the benefits of your efforts.

The relaxation produced by meditating is a powerful tool for managing stress. You learned in Chapters 1 and 2 of the many ways the body and mind react to a perceived threat. These reactions are a function of the sympathetic nervous system, which is activated in the face of perceived danger—whether real or imagined. It puts the mind and body in survival mode. Conversely, the parasympathetic nervous system activates calming, reenergizing, and other growth functions. It facilitates essential cognitive and creative processes. The parasympathetic system is responsible for stimulation of "rest-and-digest" or "feed and breed" activities that occur when the body is at rest. Meditation curtails stress by activating the parasympathetic nervous system.

The nervous system has the capacity to reverse the effects of the stress response upon entering a relaxed state. In a relaxed state, the parasympathetic nervous system is activated, as opposed to the sympathetic nervous system, which operates in stressful situations.

Although relaxation is beneficial in its own right, it can be a step in pursuit of one or more other goals. One study found that relaxation training that focused on peripheral blood flow widened peripheral blood vessels; this resulted in improved blood flow, a reduction in peripheral pain, and improved ambulation. The training, which was done in a single session, enhanced healing; individuals who took the training showed increased ability with coping skills. Recent studies suggest that relaxation training, meditation, and guided imagery can be effective for an array of self-care goals, including lowering blood glucose and A1C levels, heart rate, and blood pressure.

Some forms of meditation involve a combination of inner-focused techniques to achieve an objective. There are many ways to meditate. Three forms of meditation are presented in this chapter: *1*) basic forms of meditation, *2*) mindfulness meditation, and *3*) meditation that addresses specific troubling aspects of diabetes.

How Do I Prepare to Meditate?

Maximizing the power of meditation begins with having a positive frame for the technique. You don't have to believe you can do it, but you have to not believe that you cannot do it. In other words, it is important to begin the learning process with an open mind. The *mindful questions* are:

MQ | *Does my frame (belief) about meditation impair my ability to meditate successfully?*

What frame will get me started with meditation at my very best?

In case you are stymied on this one, how about, "Millions of people have used meditation successfully for centuries, and I can do it, too."

Next, it is essential to make a commitment to pursue the practice of meditation with enthusiasm and determination. You might do well to review the importance of commitment in Chapter 4: A Goal-Minded Approach to Behavior Change. Having an optimistic attitude and the resolve to succeed, you are ready to prepare to meditate. The principles that follow apply to any type of meditation you choose.

- Studies indicate that meditating can lower your blood glucose level. If you have any reason to think your glucose level is low, then **check your blood before starting to meditate.** Also, if you are a beginner, it would be wise to check your glucose level before and after meditating at least a few times to see its effect on your blood glucose levels.
- Select a time to practice when you will not be interrupted or distracted. Early in the morning, when the phone is not likely to ring, is usually a good time. If you try to meditate late in the day and you are tired, then you are likely to fall asleep. Eliminating any distraction is important at the start of training, but once you have learned to meditate, noise and other potential distractions will not be disturbing. It will be helpful, too, to pick a time that you can use regularly, at least at the beginning.
- Choose a comfortable place to practice. It is best to sit upright, with both feet on the floor and your hands resting on your thighs. Sitting upright does not mean sitting stiffly. Remain upright, and allow your shoulders to slacken slightly. Check your body for any tension or other discomfort, and do what you have to do to be comfortable.
- If at any time you feel uncomfortable or you need to move, stretch, or scratch, do it—do whatever you need to do to eliminate physical distractions.
- Although you might be tempted to question how you are doing, questioning whether you are doing it right or

whether it is working is contrary to your objective. Keep the practice as simple as possible; the fewer distractions the better. And if you are distracted, just let it go and return to your meditation.

- Your mind will wander, often at first. When you realize that you have lost your focus, just return to your meditation *without judgment or self-criticism.* The idea that the purpose of meditating is to still the mind is not realistic for most of us. With practice, you will be able to calm the mind's chatter, but it won't turn off completely, at least not all of the time. When you find your mind wandering, return to where you were just before you wandered, take a deep breath, and continue meditating.

- Do not try to make anything happen. Do not keep anything from happening. Simply let happen whatever happens. Meditation is an exercise in letting go physically and mentally.

- It is wise not to practice soon after eating a big meal or after consuming caffeine.

- Do not jump to conclusions if the results do not seem to be as good as you had hoped. Many who practice meditation attain a significant meditative state quickly; many others, however, require extended practice. If you need more time to practice, allow yourself that time. You deserve it. Being patient and committed to the practice will pay off. Have no doubts.

- Breathing is central to the practice of meditation, and belly breathing is the best for meditating and for your general health. Breathing "into the belly" is slower and deeper than breathing "into the chest." The latter is breathing shallowly and tends to be rapid. See the box on Belly Breathing on page 274.

- Relaxation is usually an objective in meditation because a relaxed state shuts out the distracting noise of worrisome thoughts and their undesirable consequences. In most cases, the deeper the relaxation, the better it is for achieving any other goals.

BELLY BREATHING (DIAPHRAGMATIC BREATHING)

Diaphragmatic breathing, often referred to as belly breathing, provides the lungs with the most air with the least effort. It is essential for relaxing and meditating.

Lie down on your back, placing one hand on your upper chest and the other hand on your belly just below the rib cage. Breathe in slowly through your nose. Exhale through pursed lips. As you take in a breath, is it your chest or belly that expands? Most people tend to breathe in a way that expands the chest, which is a shallow way of breathing. When the belly is expanding with each breath intake, you are getting the most air to your lungs. Belly breathing uses the diaphragm, a muscle under the lungs that separates the chest cavity from the stomach. Using the diaphragm to draw in and push out air is the most effective way to breathe. Continue to practice until it comes easily. When you get it right, your belly will rise as you breathe in and fall as you let the air out. There will not be any significant movement in your chest. It will probably be easier to learn belly breathing lying down, but it can be done in the same way in a sitting position.

Belly breathing may feel unnatural at first because most of us have been conditioned to breathe in a shallow, hurried manner. Like learning any skill, the road to success is commitment, patience, and practice. Practice at least a few minutes at a time several times a day and longer when possible, until it comes naturally and easily.

How Do I Meditate?

Three forms of meditation will be described in detail: basic, mindfulness-based stress reduction, and diabetes-specific. Some suggestions for varying the process are noted also.

BASIC MEDITATION

The first model is a classic approach that is focused on relaxing the mind and body. It is often used in combination with other forms of meditation to achieve an even deeper state of relaxation or to pursue other goals, such as building self-confidence and reducing anger or pain. Take time to become familiar with the variety of meditations presented in this chapter.

Start with the Basic Meditation. Practice it once a day, if possible, until it feels very natural. Then you might consider practicing a variation or another form to achieve a particular result. If the form of meditation you are practicing does not get easier, consider trying an alternative.

HOW TO PERFORM BASIC MEDITATION

- Sit upright in a comfortable chair, with your feet flat on the floor and your arms and hands resting on your lap. Close your eyes, unless closing them makes you uneasy. If you choose to keep your eyes open, pick a neutral spot on a wall—a spot you can comfortably focus on that does not distract you from centering your attention on your breathing.
- Take a deep breath through your nose and hold it momentarily, creating a slight tension. Then, as you exhale through pursed lips, be aware of the air and tension leaving your body altogether.
- Repeat the deep breath again. If you still feel some tension or tightness, repeat it a few more times.
- Now, breathe in and out fully and easily. Breathe in through your nose "into your belly" and exhale from your mouth. Listen to your breathing, feel your breathing, hear your breathing. Paying attention to your breathing does not mean thinking about your breathing; it means simply being aware of this rhythmic wonder of life. With each exhalation, let yourself relax. Begin to feel every part of your body letting go, every muscle coming to rest—your mind is becoming quieter and calmer.
- Breathe normally and easily, relaxing more deeply with each and every breath you take. Inhale and exhale fully. Remember, do not try to make anything happen. Do not try to keep anything from happening. Simply accept what is happening. If nothing seems to be happening, then simply experience nothing happening.
- Breathe in and breathe out. With each breath, feel yourself becoming more and more relaxed. You may choose to say to yourself with each exhalation: "relax" or "let go."

- Continue to focus on your breathing, inhaling and exhaling rhythmically, comfortably. With each exhalation, imagine that as the air flows out of your mouth, all of the tension is flowing out of your body. As you exhale, blow out all the waste and clutter that has been weighing you down. Be aware that every muscle in your body is releasing, letting go of any and all tension. Your mind is becoming calmer and quieter. As you inhale be aware of how the new air is nourishing and strengthening you physically and mentally.
- Other thoughts may come to mind. Simply go back to focusing on your breath and the deep feelings of relaxation that are filling you from head to toes.
- Continue this practice for at least 8–12 minutes, unless you are feeling uncomfortable doing it, in which case end the practice as necessary.
- To conclude the practice, count from one to five, open your eyes, and take time to reorient yourself. Gently stretch your arms and legs, smile, and give yourself a warm hug for taking good care of you. Be aware of the positive changes that have occurred with the practice.

Variations of the Basic Meditation

Counting the Breaths

Once you have begun a comfortable cycle of breathing, start counting each full breath. As you exhale, say to yourself "one." On the next exhalation, say "two," and on the next, "three." Count along with each breath. If at any time you lose track of the count, do not give it a second thought; simply start counting again with "one." Remember, the objective is to experience the process without judging or evaluating what is happening. Do everything the same as the Basic Meditation, with the addition of counting each breath. Some people find it easier to count the breaths up to 10 and then to start over at 1.

Counting Breathing Cycles

Once you have begun a comfortable cycle of breathing, begin a rhythmic count on the inhalation, starting with "one" and continuing until you have inhaled fully. As you begin to exhale, start counting from "one" until you have exhaled fully. With the next inhalation, start counting again; continue this pattern each time you inhale and exhale. A common cycle is a slow count of one to four or five on the inhalation and one to five or six on the exhalation. It is as if you are counting the length of each inhalation and exhalation. Find your cycle. When you get it right, it will feel very natural—effortless.

A Visual Meditation

This meditation adds another dimension to the process; it makes use of your imagination. It is a popular form that many have found to be very effective. It requires that you visualize a place or event that brings back your most positive memories and feelings. For some, it might be walking on the beach or walking on a wooded trail. For others, it might be a special vacation or their wedding. Make certain that you have a totally positive physical and emotional response to whatever you choose. For this step-by-step guide, we will use a walk on the beach, which should enable you to adapt the approach to any other imagery successfully.

The practice begins the same as the Basic Meditation (page 275) and/or any variation above.

- As you are feeling more and more relaxed, imagine you are at that special place that has so many positive, comforting memories for you.
- See yourself walking on a beach . . . a favorite beach. It is a beautiful day. The sun is shining brightly, and you feel the warmth over your body. You feel the wind coming off the ocean, contrasting with the heat of the sun. Feel the sand as you walk along the beach. If you are walking close to the water, the sand is wet and cool. If you are walking away from the water, the sand is dry and hot.
- Every sensation helps you relax more deeply. With every breath you take, you feel more at ease. With each exhalation, any tension or worry drains away with the exhalation.

- As you continue to walk along the beach, use all of your senses to make the experience as vivid as possible. Feel the sun, the wind, and the sand. Hear the wonderfully soothing sounds of the ocean waves. See in your mind's eye the waves rolling in to the shore, becoming white and bubbly as the water rolls along the sand and then begins the return back to the ocean. Perhaps you can hear or see some seagulls. Perhaps some children are making a sand-castle, and you can hear their chatter and laughter.
- Every muscle is letting go, coming to rest. Your mind is more and more calm and quiet. A deep sense of inner peace and ease is filling you completely.
- If you find yourself wandering away from the beach scene, just gently take yourself back there without any judgment or self-criticism. The only thought that is needed is "Oh, I have wandered. OK. Now back to the beach."
- Use all of your senses to make the image of the beach as vivid as possible. Hear the sounds and see the sights that you know so well from memories of being there. With each experience, let go; let yourself relax more deeply. Your arms and legs and your entire body may feel pleas-antly heavy, sinking into where you are sitting. Or you may feel very light, as if you are floating. Remember, don't try to make anything happen or keep anything from happening. When you let go, it will happen the way you need it to happen.
- Deep, deep relaxation . . . all your muscles are relaxed, at ease. Your mind is calm and quiet.
- Continue to walk on the beach for as long as you want. Know that when you end this practice, you will continue to feel relaxed but alert and fully prepared to deal with anything that you need to do. You will feel a renewed energy. You will feel mentally stronger. You will feel a pleasant sense of accomplishment.
- When you are ready to stop, blank out the image of the beach. Let go of the image of the beach with a smile, knowing that you can come back to it at any time you

choose. Count from one to five, and gently open your eyes. Take a few moments to reorient yourself to time and place. Stretch and now do whatever makes sense for you to do, feeling strong and enthusiastic with every endeavor. Be sure to give yourself a big hug for taking good care of you.

Variations of the Visual Meditation

Changing the Scene

You can use any scene that is positive. Follow the same general style as described above. If your special place is a walk on a mountain trail, use your memories of that experience to activate each of your senses, so that the imagery is as vivid as possible. The objective is to become as absorbed in the scene as possible.

See the trees and wildflowers, perhaps stopping to lean closer and smell them. Hear the sound of the wind rustling the leaves and the sound of birds and of other small creatures scampering through the woods. Hear the sound of your footsteps, the crack of a small branch that you stepped on. See the stream or lake (if one is not in your special place, you can create one) and all of the stimuli that are common to it. As you focus on the details of the scene, be aware of becoming more and more relaxed, and more and more at ease.

Creative Imagery

It is not necessary to use imagery that is based on a past experience. Another form of meditation, sometimes referred to as "creative visualization," is to construct a scene that is of your choosing, based on some particular objective. For example, many people who struggle with anxiety have used this form to create a "safe house," a place they can go to in their mind's eye where it is comfortable, pleasant, and totally safe.

Your safe house can be on the beach or at the top of a mountain. It can be a cave or in the sky. Having chosen a place, create a structure . . . your dream home or something out of science fiction. Is it a log cabin, a castle, or a fortress? Is it round, square, or rectangular? Is it underground or on a mountain-top? Every detail is yours to choose; make it as comfortable and appealing as you can.

Then paint the walls, hang some pictures, and furnish it. Let each step of the way help you relax . . . more and more deeply with each new detail. Keep in mind that you can do anything you want in this process so long as the end result is feeling safe.

Once you have created your safe house, use your senses to help you stay focused and relaxed. Visualize the setting you have created. Enjoy your creation in every detail. If there are windows and a view, see and enjoy it; feel the peace and calmness it brings to you. Hear your favorite music, and smell your favorite smells (is your favorite pie baking?). With each breath and with each sensory detail, feel your body relax more deeply, with your mind becoming more quiet and calm.

End this practice as you would end the Basic Meditation (see page 275), knowing that you can go to your safe place at any time to relax and let go of tension and anxiety by repeating this meditation. Once you have created your safe place and it is familiar to you, you need only go directly there to enjoy its comforts and safety.

Another Example of Creative Imagery

As you focus on your breath, imagine that the air entering your body has the quality of light. See your body slowly filling with light. It can be entering your body with your breath or it can be entering through the pores in your skin. Just let the light enter and fill you. It can be entering through the top of your head or your feet. Be creative. The light can be daylight, lamplight, or a magical glow. You can give it any color that pleases you. You might experiment with allowing the light to enter one part of your body at a time or simply letting it fill your body in no particular order. (I prefer starting with the face and head; then down into the neck and shoulders; next the arms, hands, and fingers; then my chest and lower torso; and finally my legs, feet, and toes.) As the light enters each part of your body, feel that part becoming more and more relaxed. If you sense tension in a specific part of your body, breathe the light to that part and feel it becoming relaxed and letting go of the strain. (In my practice, I see the light as healing each part of my body.)

Building Self-Confidence

A visual meditation can help build confidence. In the meditative state, the mind is more elastic and more susceptible to positive suggestions. If increasing your confidence is a goal, add this self-affirmation to the meditation you are practicing: "Day by day in every way, I feel stronger and stronger . . . more confident in my ability to do what I have to do to get where I want to be. Day by day, I am finding my voice, which means I am less and less susceptible to the voices of others, especially of others who are not good for me. Day by day, I am increasingly aware of my worth." As you recite these positive statements, see yourself standing tall, strong, and confident. You can repeat this passage as often as you want during a meditation practice.

Releasing Anger

A visual meditation can be used to relieve angry feelings. As you learned in Chapter 6: Essential People Skills, keeping anger in control is essential to keeping stress in check. Meditation practice can help control anger in two ways: 1) by using the technique to shift from feeling angry to feeling calm and relaxed and 2) by discharging welled-up antagonism by way of an imaginary emotional release.

A colleague told me many years ago that when she was angry she would buy a large rump roast, take it into the woods, and pulverize it with a baseball bat, imagining that the piece of meat was the source of her disdain. Of course, that was back when the cost of that hunk of meat was much less than today, but the point is well taken—doing something symbolic can have the desired effect without doing something inappropriate like pulverizing someone in reality. Creative meditation can be helpful with anger management. If you imagine pulverizing someone or something, it can have the same unburdening results as actually doing it, without any of the unpleasant consequences . . . or financial burden.

Start with the Basic Meditation (page 275) to become physically and mentally relaxed. When you have reached that good place, add the following component (or a variation that better suits you) to your practice. Imagine that you are walking along a wooded trail. As you follow the trail around a bend, you see a large boulder in your path. You approach the rock and notice that there is a sledgehammer nearby. You may want to associate the rock with someone or with a particular issue, but you are likely to find the exercise just as helpful by seeing the boulder as a representation of your anger in general. Pick up the hammer, and start to pulverize the boulder. See yourself pounding the object with intense passion. Feel it; hear it as vividly as possible. If necessary, take a break from hammering the rock to rest and recharge; then return to the task at hand. When you have reduced the boulder to a pile of pebbles, put the hammer down and proceed with the energizing, soothing part of the practice. Focus on your breathing and the deep sense of inner peace and satisfaction within. See yourself walking along the wooded trail, or any other specific scene you have created, feeling lighter and more content. You feel deeply relaxed and at peace—your body is relaxed and energized. If, for any reason, obvious or not, this part of the practice is too upsetting, then discontinue it and focus on your breathing and any other safe and calming imagery.

For the reader who has access to the Internet, there are numerous websites and apps that present a wide range of ways to meditate and ways to enhance the experience with sound (ocean waves, gongs and Tibetan bells, music) and visual imagery (ocean waves, sunsets, graphics that represent relaxed breathing). Use your search engine or your App Store to search "meditation."

Mindfulness-Based Stress Reduction (MBSR) Versus Living Mindfully

MBSR

The core of MBSR is the practice of meditation to systematically train the body and mind to be in the present and to be fully aware of what is happening internally and externally. Mindful meditation is a fully present, nonreactive, and nonjudgmental awareness of the moment. It is being attentive without distorting reality with personal feelings, prejudices, or interpretations. The training engenders a refinement of attention and awareness, compassion, and wisdom.

Mindfulness-based meditation shifts the mind from a mode of self-talk based on one's conscious and unconscious beliefs and biases to an objective modality in which the focus is on one's thoughts, feelings, and sensations over time. It is a shift from mindless self-acceptance to being nonjudgmentally curious about who and what we are.

Mindfulness meditation will not be the "answer" to all of your problems, but it can enable you to clearly see those problems without the noise and disarray of a cluttered mind, and with that clarity, provide a reasonable chance of resolving most problems.

Having conducted MBSR training for several decades, the University of Massachusetts Medical School's Center for Mindfulness reports that as the ability to be mindfully present grows, the practitioners become more relaxed, patient, compassionate, forgiving, and happier people. Life goes more smoothly, they are less stressed out, relationships with others improve, life's little blessings are enjoyed more, and they don't sweat the small stuff as much.

With more than three decades of scientific research at various medical centers, there is evidence to suggest that training in mindfulness and MBSR can positively, and often profoundly, reduce medical symptoms and psychological distress. Studies have shown that MBSR can be an effective complement to the treatment of a range of maladies, including anxiety, cancer, substance abuse disorders, chronic pain, diabetes, fibromyalgia, gastrointestinal disorders, heart disease, depression, and stress disorders. It should be noted, however, that many of these studies concluded that further research was needed to substantiate the findings.

LIVING MINDFULLY

Living mindfully is bringing all aspects of MBSR into daily life (see Chapter 3: Being Mindful). The process in daily life involves taking moments throughout the day to pause and be present, to take a moment to feel and observe yourself breathing. Mindful living is tuning in to the present and what is happening inside and out, not only when meditating but also when you are living day to day. It is being mindful when you eat, walk, or have a conversation; it is being aware with compassion and wisdom in all your activities.

Living mindfully brings to awareness our natural inclination to become attached to our beliefs about ourselves and the world around us—even when they have no basis in reality and, even worse, when they are distressing or self-destructive. With this awareness, the practitioner is able to *let go* of faulty beliefs (frames, thoughts, and assumptions). Letting go is fundamental to the practice of mindfulness (see Chapter 9: The Frame of Letting Go).

Being mindful allows us to distinguish between a subjective and an objective interpretation of our experiences. To perceive something objectively is to see it in the same way as anyone else would see it. Carson had an episode of hypoglycemia, her blood glucose level was severely low, and she passed out. Anyone who witnessed the event would agree that she lost consciousness, and anyone who saw her blood glucose level and understood diabetes would concur that her low level of glucose caused her to faint. However, a subjective interpretation of the same event by two or more individuals can be extremely diverse. William may see the event from a critical perspective:

"Carson is reckless and that's why this happened." Lily has compassion for her friend and criticizes the parents for not providing Carson with a continuous glucose monitor that probably would have prevented the problem.

MBSR Meditation

Begin the practice of MBSR with an open mind that is absent of assumptions or expectations about the outcome. In Kabat-Zinn's seminal book on mindfulness (*Full Catastrophe Living: Using the Wisdom of Your Body and Mind to Face Stress, Pain, and Illness* [16]), it is noted that participants in their MBSR classes do the best with the attitude, "I don't know whether this will work or not and I have my doubts, but I am going to give it my best shot and see what happens."

FUNDAMENTALS

MBSR meditation is about *observing yourself objectively*, simply witnessing what is happening without analyzing or judging what you behold. It is being aware of where your attention is moment to moment. Imagine your objective observer is an alter-ego, a second self whose only mission is to help you meditate. Its only interest is to remind you to return to meditating when you have wandered from it—worrying about being able to meditate, thinking about tasks to be done or a problem at work or your next meal. Acceptance is essential. If your mind wanders—and it will—your objective self doesn't say you are bad or stupid; it merely reminds you to return to the pure state of *being* without the need of *doing* anything else. Imagine the relief that comes with moments in which you are free from having to do anything, including thinking about what has happened or what might happen.

It is essential to practice regularly, every day if possible, and preferably at the same time. These are guidelines for a beginner. In time, and with regular practice, you will be able to meditate anywhere, including in a New York subway train.

THE PRACTICE

1. **Set a time limit.** If you're just beginning, it might help to choose a short time, such as 5 or 10 minutes. Also, set an alarm as a signal to end the practice—preferably one that is gentle in tone.

2. **Find a relaxed, comfortable position.** You could be seated on a chair or on the floor on a cushion. If you choose to sit on the floor, there is no need to cross your legs in an attempt to depict the inimitable Buddha. Whether you are in a chair or on the floor, make certain that you are comfortable. If you feel uncomfortable at any time, do what is necessary to eliminate whatever is bothering you.

3. **Close your eyes.** Your mind will be active enough without the distraction of what you might see. If keeping your eyes closed causes you uneasiness, pick a neutral place in your line of vision to focus on, such as a scratch in the paint on a wall.

4. **Focus on your breathing.** You won't find this step in many renditions of mindful meditation, but I have been meditating for over 30 years. I have trained in MBSR and have found tuning into the breath very effective in getting centered in the moment. Feel the natural flow of breath—in and out. You don't need to do anything to your breath, just breathe naturally. When one breath ends, the next breath begins. (See How to Perform Basic Meditation on pages 275–276.)

5. **Observe the present moment as it is.** Remember, the aim of mindfulness is not quieting the mind or attempting to achieve a state of either eternal calm or cosmic consciousness. Just pay attention to the present moment, without judgment.

6. **Let go of anything else.** When you become aware of anything other than the moment, let it go. Although it might raise the eyebrows of some MBSR "experts,"

THE MINDFUL GUIDE TO MANAGING DIABETES

I smile as I return to the moment. It is my way of avoiding the trap of taking myself too seriously.

7. **Return to observing the present moment as it is.** Our minds often get carried away in thought. That's why mindfulness is the practice of returning, again and again, to the present moment.

8. **End the practice by returning to your breathing.** When you hear the signal to end the exercise or when you decide to stop, take a minute or two to focus on your breath.

9. **Open your eyes and smile** as you give yourself a hug for being on the way to achieving the ability to live mindfully, a powerful means of minimizing the stress in your life and enhancing your proficiency with regard to managing your diabetes.

Celebrate a fact: you are keeping a commitment to train in this very doable and highly valuable procedure. Give no attention to speculating on or making assumptions about the future. Before your next practice session, ask these *mindful questions*:

MQ | *Reflecting on my last practice, was there any distraction that was difficult to let go of?*

Without giving the matter undue attention, can I figure out why it was a problem?

What could I do to make the next practice more effective? Position myself more comfortably? Shorten the time I meditate? Give the identified distraction a humorous name or image to dispel whatever hold it had on my practice?

As is the case for general meditative principles and practices, there is an abundance of websites and apps dedicated to mindfulness meditation and MBSR. Use either title to search for additional guidance.

Diabetes-Specific Meditation

Unfortunately, meditation cannot rid you of diabetes. But meditating regularly can help you deal with it more easily, with less discomfort, and with a greater sense of empowerment. The practice of meditation can help manage the stress of diabetes in many ways. It can reduce the experience of pain, build confidence and self-esteem, and help you overcome irrational fear.

Start with the Basic Meditation (page 275) to achieve physical and mental calmness. Feeling relaxed, choose one of the following meditations to achieve a specific objective.

MODERATING PAIN

Give each segment of the meditation as much time as needed to fully capture the imagery. Let go of any preconceived notions. Allow yourself to see and feel the changes being suggested.

When you feel relaxed by practicing the Basic Meditation (page 275), focus your attention on the part of your body where you want to ease the pain. For example, if your feet hurt, see them in your mind's eye as clearly as possible. Begin to see the area that hurts as being red, the color most associated with heat. Imagine that the pain has the physical quality of redness. Stay with this image until it is very clear.

Now, imagine that with each inhalation, the air entering your body has the color of cool, light blue (or any other color you choose, so long as it has a soothing, cooling quality). Once the image of a blue light entering your body with each breath is well established, begin to imagine sending that light to your feet. See the bluish air entering your body and going to your feet. With each breath, imagine the cool, light blue air going to the painful areas. See that the redness is gradually getting lighter and lighter, from red to pink and then even lighter. Begin to see the areas you are focusing on changing to a cool light blue. (If you had a can of red paint and continually added a light blue paint to the can, the red would steadily get lighter, becoming more pinkish, until it was the color of blue you were adding.) As the redness diminishes, the pain lessens. With each breath and with the steady flow of cool, blue air to the area of your choice, you feel more comfortable and more at ease. As the target area becomes totally blue, there is no pain or there is so little discomfort that it does not matter. Stay with this imagery as long you desire.

When you are ready to stop, blank out the imagery, count from one to five, and gently open your eyes. Take time to reorient yourself to time and place. Gently stretch your arms and legs, smile, and give yourself a congratulatory hug. Now, fully alert, do what you want to do, feeling strong, comfortable, and content.

EASING FEAR OF COMPLICATIONS

Give each segment of the meditation as much time as needed to fully capture the imagery. When you feel relaxed by practicing the Basic Meditation (page 275), begin to see yourself in a very special place, a place that feels invigorating and inspirational. (See Creative Imagery on page 279 for some ideas.) Envision a place that is as beautiful as you can imagine, as safe and as comfortable as your imagination can conjure. It can be real or completely made up. Make it a place where you are totally protected from unwelcome intrusion: a fort on a mountain top, a satellite orbiting earth, a yellow submarine. Having chosen your special place, develop the image in fine detail. In this process, let yourself become even more deeply relaxed. See yourself there looking at the surroundings both near and far, using all of your senses to make the vision as vivid and imposing as possible.

When the scene is vivid in your imagination, recite these words: "Day by day, I am stronger and more confident. I believe

I am capable of doing everything I need to do to manage my diabetes and prevent the onset of complications. I know my situation is not the same as anyone in the past who had endured serious consequences from diabetes. I have strengths, knowledge, and resources that those in the past did not have. With each breath, with each day, I am stronger and stronger, more and more confident that I can and will do what is needed to keep my blood glucose levels in a healthy range most of the time. As I live more and more mindfully, I feel a new power that is energizing and gratifying. When I have a momentary setback, I will smile and seize the opportunity to turn the misfortune in a positive direction. I take diabetes seriously. I respect diabetes. I do not fear it. Each moment I am in my special place, I feel more invigorated and more confident. A deep sense of courage fills me."

Repeat these words or any part of them at least once as you continue to see yourself in your special place. Feel an inner strength growing with each breath, each image, and each thought. Know that you can and will do what is necessary to minimize the risk of complications.

When you are ready to stop, blank out the image of your special place, count from one to five, and gently open your eyes. Take a few moments to reorient yourself to time and place. Gently stretch and then proceed with doing what you want to do, feeling strong, enthusiastic, and wonderfully optimistic about the future. Remember to give yourself a big hug for taking good care of you.

REDUCING PAIN FROM POOR PERIPHERAL BLOOD FLOW

In a study noted earlier in this chapter, patients who suffered from narrowed peripheral blood vessels experienced significant relief by learning to relax at will. The aim of the training was to raise the temperature of the feet, which, in turn, widened the blood vessels and allowed an increase in blood flow.

When you feel relaxed by practicing the Basic Meditation, focus your attention on your feet. Now, create an image that is likely to warm them. For example, you might see your feet soaking in warm water. Picture this image in your mind's eye as vividly as possible. Feel the warmth of the water as it warms and soothes every part of your feet: your toes, soles, insteps, and ankles. Imagine the perfect environment surrounding you. Everything is pleasant and comfortable to the eye and ear. (Some people use recordings of the sounds of ocean waves or a gentle rain to help to relax.) Imagine that as your feet absorb the warmth, your blood vessels are expanding, letting in more warmth and releasing any discomfort. Continue this pattern of imagining greater warmth and slighter discomfort. Imagine the vessels that supply blood to your feet widening and allowing more blood to flow through each foot.

IMPROVING PERFORMANCE

Many athletes use meditation to enhance their performance. The practice of meditation allows athletes to overcome faults by rehearsing the proper execution of their sport. For example, a baseball player who tends to be impatient and swings at bad pitches might meditate on letting any pitch in a specific zone go by. Also, the practice enables the athlete to prepare mentally for any possible event. One of the common ways for an athlete or an athletic team to lose is to be caught off guard by the opponent's strategy. To avoid being blindsided, the athlete might meditate on various possible scenarios. Preparing for a tennis match with an opponent who is not known for a strong backhand, a competitor might meditate on the possibility that his rival has developed his backhand (envisioning seeing his opponent displaying a powerful backhand), so he won't be caught short if it happens. The effort required for good diabetes management has similarities to athletic performance.

Identify an aspect of diabetes care that has been difficult for you. Then, identify what behavior you need to initiate to eliminate the problem. For example, you may need to be more effective in asserting your issues when you see your physician and other care providers. In this case, you would rehearse being more assertive than usual, playing out scenes in which you are assertively telling your provider what you need from the consultation, making certain that the important issues get addressed. Another example is going to a party where you won't know many people. You can use the power of meditation to anticipate some scenarios that might be unfavorable and to practice positive ways that you can respond if such events occur. End this practice the same way as any other meditation exercise.

Adding Power Self-Affirmations

Self-affirmations are statements or declarations made to oneself to encourage and support you in life's endeavors. Making self-validating statements is a technique that has been used successfully by individuals recovering from substance abuse and other addictions. The idea is to program the mind and body with positive messages that build confidence and optimistic outcomes. As we have said many times and in many ways, what you believe is central to what you do. Positive self-affirmations reinforce positive beliefs and replace negative beliefs with repetition. Here are some examples of power self-affirmations:

- "I am capable of doing everything I need to do to manage my diabetes well."
- "I can and will say no to anything that jeopardizes my diabetes management."
- "Everything is not the way I want it, but I still have so much to be grateful for."
- "I will not be hard on myself today, even if I stumble."
- "My purpose is to live well with diabetes. I deserve it!"

While meditating, and at any other time, recite one or more self-affirmations.

What If I Can't Meditate?

You can meditate. If you are committed to learning to meditate and it has not worked, there are two possibilities: *1*) you have not found the type of meditation that will work for you or *2*) your effort is being blocked by a glitch, probably in your expectations. Give the meditation you have chosen a reasonable trial.

Keep in mind that your thinking will drift in many directions: to the past or future, to wondering if the practice is "working," to questioning your ability to meditate. Accept these distractions as an opportunity to develop your awareness and your ability to return to the present without needing to analyze or judge what happened.

FINDING WHAT WORKS FOR YOU

In this chapter, there are detailed descriptions of various ways to meditate. Each of the meditations has been used extensively and with considerable success. However, as you practice any one of them, you may have a sense that some variation would be better for you. If so, give your version a try. There is no absolute way to meditate. There are so many ways to achieve a meditative state; the one that is right is the one that works for you. Just keep in mind the principles of meditation that were described earlier, and create a script that works. Be creative. Experiment until you find the right script for you.

For example, if focusing on your breath does not work, consider focusing your attention initially on a specific, neutral place within your vision. You might select an object in the room or a spot on the wall. Make certain that it does not distract from your objective. Simply focus your attention on this inactive spot or object. Focusing on a burning candle—real or imagined—can be mesmerizing. Another possibility is to envision a vacation or other experience you have had that was very positive. See the experience in as much detail as possible as you let yourself relax more deeply with the imagery. Focusing on your breathing is simple, and, for many, it is both easy and magical.

If you had to stop because you were uncomfortable, take some time to reflect on why you were not at ease. The *mindful questions* are:

MQ | *What made me uneasy?*

Was it something specific to the practice or to unrelated circumstances?

Would one of the variations help me become more focused and at ease during the practice?

It might be helpful to record or have someone record the procedure. Some people respond better to being guided by an audio presentation of the meditation process.

ELIMINATING BARRIERS

A common barrier to meditating successfully is having a negative frame about meditation. The *mindful question* is:

MQ | *What frame or frames do I have about meditation that are working against my being successful?*

Some examples are: "I can't meditate." "I would have to sit for a long time like a statue and in an awkward position, which is not appealing." "It is mystical and that bothers me." "I will lose control." None of these frames is real. Each one requires mindful reframing.

Another obstacle to look for is unrealistic expectations about the experience. For many beginners, the practice can be frustrating because it can be difficult to maintain focus on the breath or whatever thoughts and images are being used to achieve a meditative state. The challenge is to recognize that your attention has wandered off course and to simply return to where you want to be without judgment. You will wander—more at the beginning than when you have practiced for a while. When you do, simply refocus over and over without judging the process or yourself. Remember (from Chapter 10) that any frame with "should" in it is a problem. The frame, "I should be getting deeply relaxed by now" or "I shouldn't be wandering again" will hamper your ability to accomplish your goal.

Another stumbling block is to have false expectations about meditation and the meditative state. It is neither an unconscious state nor a mystical experience. It might feel trance-like, but you will not be asleep or in a stupor, unresponsive to what is going on in your world. If the phone rings, you will hear it and have to choose whether or not to answer it. If something requires your urgent attention, you will react accordingly. You are never out of control.

MAINTAINING MOTIVATION

You can meditate and enjoy its many benefits. Certainly, some individuals will have more difficulty mastering the technique, but the effort will pay off in the end, even if it is a struggle getting started. Even if nothing seems to be happening at first, the fact that you have made a commitment and you are steadfast in pursuing it is progress. If you continue to have difficulty, it might help to get into a problem-solving mode (see Chapter 11). Also, on page 271, revisit How Do I Prepare to Meditate? Finally, look again for internal barriers, such as a negative frame about meditating, that might be preventing you from fully entering the meditative state.

If you are hesitant about committing the time to meditation, review the list of benefits at the beginning of the chapter to see what your rewards will be. Once you are meditating regularly, the benefits will be phenomenal.

PART 4

Type 1 Diabetes

CHAPTER 16

Stress and Type 1 Diabetes

The diagnosis of type 1 diabetes in childhood marks the beginning of a lifetime of challenges for everyone involved. While type 1 diabetes can develop at any age, this chapter focuses on the numerous sources of stress in raising a child with the disease. The regimen for managing the disease will permeate every aspect of a child's life. For the parents and family, the problems may feel unbearably endless. How does a family deal with the fact that their child has a chronic and potentially life-threatening disease? How does the child— infancy to the teens—cope with his or her condition?

Although type 1 diabetes can be extremely difficult, it does not have to be an endlessly burdensome ordeal. With knowledgeable parents who are patient and compassionate, along with a network of support from family, friends, and healthcare professionals, most children with type 1 diabetes not only survive, they thrive. (For practical reasons, "parents" will be designated as the primary care providers; the term may refer to the child's grandparents, foster parents, or whomever is raising the youngster.)

Let's not sugarcoat a serious and sometimes excruciating situation for all parties concerned. But, starting strong—with the right tools and resources—the journey will be much less difficult. Starting from weakness will make what is already difficult extremely stressful and dangerous.

Stress is a nemesis to diabetes management. When the patient is a child, the ensuing problems can be very stressful.

Common causes of stress when coping with type 1 diabetes are lack of knowledge, intense and/or uncontrolled emotions, and inadequate support. In this chapter, the stressors that parents and others may experience when their child is diagnosed with diabetes are considered from various perspectives: the parents, the child, siblings, and an array of others who might be involved with the youngster. A range of likely causes of stress are identified along with ways to eliminate or, at least, minimize them. Here and throughout the book, the power of *mindfulness* is used to resolve conflicts and other problems.

Sources of Stress for Parents Raising a Child With Type 1 Diabetes

CHALLENGE: LACK OF KNOWLEDGE

Picture someone balancing on a high wire while juggling five bowling pins. The image is analogous to the difficulties a parent faces raising a toddler with type 1 diabetes. The juggler has knowledge of differences in wire tension, of balance, and of what can cause a mishap. Perhaps most importantly, the performer perfects his act through endless practice. Parents will get lots of practice, but they first must learn what to do and how to do it.

Most hospitals have pediatric units and pediatric specialists to provide training in the basics for managing the disease, including insulin injection technique, blood glucose monitoring, appropriate infant feeding, and recognition and treatment of hypoglycemia and hyperglycemia. It is essential to have a pediatric specialist involved in a child's care. If this service is not immediately available, ask your doctors for information about programs that might be available nearby. Also, the Internet can be a valuable resource for information and support (although, please note that the Internet is neither a substitute for visits with your healthcare team nor does it take the place of diabetes education from a pediatric specialist). In Chapter 14, various ways of using the Web are explored along with concerns about the validity of these sites. For example, the "Find an Education Program" tab on diabeteseducator.org lists 2,441 accredited programs throughout the United States.

From diabetes.org, you can obtain a free copy of *The Type 1 Diabetes Self-Care Manual*, which includes the basics of dealing with the condition along with a range of special considerations such as the needs of different age-groups. On this same website, there is a link to "New to Type 1 Diabetes?", where a Courage-Wisdom-Hope Kit is offered for free. The kit includes guides for parents, kids, and siblings and a few trinkets that could be very handy.

A consistently effective and efficient way to solve most problems is to approach them mindfully (see Chapter 3: Being Mindful). Mindfulness begins with a pause and one or more deep breaths depending on the degree of urgency, confusion, or fear of failure you are experiencing. This process is called centering, which means to calm your emotions and slow your mind and your breathing to a point where you can feel a lot more going on around and inside you.

Once centered, the next step is to ask the relevant *mindful questions*. With regard to being fully knowledgeable about managing the disease, ask these questions:

MQ | *Given that knowing as much as possible about diabetes management is critical to my child's well-being, what steps do I need to take to achieve this end?*

How can my child's medical team help in this regard?

Does a nearby hospital or clinic have an educational program?

Is there a support group for care providers of children with type 1 diabetes that I can join?

Is there a reliable website that provides the information I need?

From the answers to these questions, write a plan of action listing prospective contacts, phone numbers, and the specific information you are seeking.

Note: Medicare will pay for diabetes education if it is prescribed by a physician, a certified registered nurse practitioner (CRNP), or a physician assistant (PA).

CHALLENGE: URGENT DIABETIC CONDITIONS

It is imperative to know that certain conditions require immediate attention, particularly hypoglycemia (low blood glucose). If steps aren't taken to normalize a severe low blood glucose level, it can result in seizures, loss of consciousness, or death. Blood glucose levels that are either too high (hyperglycemia) or too low for too long may cause various serious conditions, including becoming comatose.

If a child has become ill, someone should contact the youngster's medical team immediately for guidance and professional oversight. Also, a person with diabetes should not be left alone when ill. For teenagers or young adults who are living away from home, it is imperative to have someone acting on their behalf when they are sick. Not being able to eat properly puts added stress on the body, which can rapidly affect blood glucose levels and may lead to a life-threatening emergency. Severe blood glucose levels can quickly impair the individual's ability to implement self-care, which is why someone must care for an individual with diabetes who has the flu or another ailment.

There is nothing more stressful than being confronted with a medical emergency and not knowing what to do. It is

TREATING A CHILD WITH HYPOGLYCEMIA

Anyone caring for a child with diabetes must know the symptoms of hypoglycemia and how to treat it. Specific treatment for a low blood glucose level should be determined by your child's age, health, and medical history. See page 59 for a list of common symptoms of low blood glucose.

For children with diabetes, the goal of treatment is to maintain a safe blood glucose level. This step involves testing blood glucose often, learning to recognize oncoming symptoms, and treating the condition quickly, based on instructions given by your child's doctor.

To treat low blood glucose immediately, your child should eat or drink something that has sugar in it, such as ornage juice, milk, cake icing, or a hard candy. Then, continue to check blood glucose levels every 15–20 minutes until they are above 100 mg/dL

---

imperative to know the signs and symptoms of a developing crisis to avert a serious, even life-threatening, situation. And if an emergency is unavoidable, knowing how to respond is essential. It is a fact: the more the family knows about diabetes, the more effective they will be in caring for the child, and the less stressful it will be for everyone. The *mindful questions* are:

MQ | *Have I been adequately informed about conditions that require immediate action?*

Do I know how to respond to a diabetic emergency?

CHALLENGE: DEALING WITH INTENSE EMOTIONS

Raising a child from infancy through adolescence can be very demanding at times. When the child has diabetes, the trying times can be unrelenting. Parents will face numerous problems that will trigger intense feelings. Caring for a child with diabetes requires changes in routines, in diet, and in lifestyle, any of which can be a source of conflict within the family. Young children with diabetes may not understand what they are being told to do regarding their care protocol, and this can result in frustration and stress for everyone concerned. Older children with the disease may be distracted from what they need to do or they might be expressing frustration-related defiance. Unwanted feelings can be aroused by the one with the condition or anyone connected to that person.

Early on, parents and other close relatives are likely to experience one or more intense emotions: fear, guilt, and depression are common. If any of the care providers has known someone with diabetes who endured serious complications, they are likely to feel intense dread. It can be very distressing when understandable concerns are intensified by false beliefs. For example, parents might assume that the child will suffer the same dreadful complications that another member of the family had endured. This assumption denies two facts: 1) the knowledge base and medical technology are much more advanced now than even a few years ago and 2) it is unlikely that there is significant commonality between these individuals— internally or externally. The belief that the circumstances are similar is without merit.

Anxiety is commonplace. There is the tale of the "helicopter mom" who hovers over her child, watching every move, as she smothers her offspring with a feverish rant of directions and criticism. This behavior is not surprising given the complexity of diabetes management in the context of an infant, a toddler, preschooler, preteen, or teenager. For some adults, the task of calibrating the amount of insulin to inject or calculating carbo-hydrates can be unnerving. Another trigger for uneasiness is when the child is at school or a sleepover. Even when their adolescent goes off to college, parents may experience consid-erable anxiety. Another source of dread is the threats posed by the disease—serious complications and severe low or high blood glucose levels, perils that can span a lifetime. The *mindful questions* are:

MQ
> *Being anxious is understandable, but am I overreacting?*
>
> *What beliefs are making me so fearful? Are they based in reality?*
>
> *Excessive stress and anxiety may impair my ability to do what is needed. Should I consult with my doctor or engage a counselor?*

CHALLENGE: FEELING GUILTY

Another problem arises when the parents of a child diagnosed with diabetes are racked with feelings of guilt. The exact cause of type 1 diabetes is not known. Generally, the body's immune system mistakenly destroys the insulin-producing cells in the pancreas. Genetics and some viruses may contribute to onset of the disease. Even if the ailment had seemingly been passed on genetically, the notion of fault is unjust. The *mindful questions* are:

MQ
> *Is there any sound basis for believing I am the cause of my child's diabetes?*
>
> *Even if my family history suggested that it was possible my newborn could develop the disease, how could I have stopped it from happening?*
>
> *Is taking responsibility for what goes wrong (self-blaming) typical for me?*

CHALLENGE: OVERCOMING FEELINGS OF SADNESS

Checking blood glucose and injecting a toddler or preschool child time and again can induce intense feelings of sadness and depression. For some parents, feelings of hopelessness tear at their faith and deepen their state of dejection. Injecting a child can be stressful, at least initially. However, if negative feelings persist and/or intensify, the suffering may signal the need for support in overcoming the problem. The *mindful questions* are:

MQ | *Who would likely be able to help me deal with these feelings? Our pediatrician? Nurse educator? Members of my support group? A professional counselor?*

Given the youth's age, would an insulin pump or a continuous glucose monitoring device help to reduce these distressing emotions?

CHALLENGE: DEALING WITH ANGER

Anger, perhaps intense at times, may be triggered by the diagnosis and subsequent journey of caring for a child with type 1 diabetes. Struggling to manage the child's blood glucose level can be scary and frustrating. Not getting a prompt or satisfying response from a doctor can be irritating. When stress levels are high, susceptibility to strong feelings can escalate.

If a child mismanages the protocol for self-care, blame and anger are common reactions. Whether the blame is directed at oneself or the youngster, it is almost always without basis. Despite the seriousness and frightfulness of the incident, it is important that the caregiver's feelings are contained. You might be tempted to punish the child, but punishment is not likely to be warranted, and it does not have a lasting effect on a child's diabetes-related behavior. Keep in mind that the capability for self-care changes throughout the development years as do some of the demands of the disease, such as an increased demand for insulin due to puberty. Research indicates that parental warmth, contracting for diabetes-related behavior, and family problem solving are effective strategies for attaining behavior changes related to diabetes.

If you have trouble controlling your temper, you need to have a plan for calming yourself down (see Chapter 5: Being Emotionally Smart). It is certainly a time for *mindful* reflection. The ***mindful questions*** are:

MQ | *What are the triggers for my becoming over-reactive?*

What is the signal to put my plan in place?

What is my plan? Meditating? Taking a walk? Praying? Calling "time out"?

How often do I plan to practice?

Do I need professional assistance?

CHALLENGE: HANDLING STRESS

At the least, intense emotions are distressing; at worst, they can be physically and/or mentally harmful for everyone concerned. Caregivers and the child are in jeopardy. Type 1 diabetes requires considerable planning, preparation, and execution, which, in turn, necessitates focus, stability, and sound thinking. Dealing with considerable stress can strongly hamper the best of intentions. Stress drains the mind and body, enhancing the risk of not doing what is required or not doing it right.

The objective is not to quell emotional reactions. In fact, trying to bottle up your feelings not only doesn't work, it will make you even more agitated. A healthy response to troubling emotions is to pause and focus on what you are feeling and to calm down so that you can respond to the situation *mindfully* (see Chapter 5: Being Emotionally Smart and Chapter 15: Mindful Meditation Plus).

Being both diabetes savvy and emotionally smart is vital. The following *mindful questions* will help you avoid acting wrongly on your feelings:

MQ | *Is there reason to believe that my emotions could impede my ability to provide proper care?*

What might trigger an undesirable emotional reaction in the context of my child's diabetes?

When I get overly emotional, what is my plan for calming down? Should I call a timeout and take a walk or briefly meditate?

What belief is driving the feeling? Is the belief rooted in fact or assumption? Is it based on my self-critical nature?

Do I need to talk to someone about my feelings? Do I need professional help?

CHALLENGE: TRANSFERRING RESPONSIBILITY

One of the most difficult decisions for parents is when to transfer responsibility for managing the disease from themselves to the child. Unfortunately, there are no clear rules to follow. Turning over responsibility even for one piece of diabetes care requires careful consideration. Transferring elements of diabetes care to a youngster who is not yet capable of such behavior—either intellectually, physically, emotionally, or mentally—will result in failure of the intended regimen, with dangerous consequences.

Answers to the following **mindful questions** may be enough to make a sound decision. However, the matter requires keen insight; it might be wise to consult with the child's medical team before deciding what to do.

MQ | *Is the child's age and cognitive level sufficient for the task?*

In most cases, the decision is intuitive. However, if you have serious doubts or your intuition appears to have been wrong, a professional opinion would be proper.

MQ | *Is his or her knowledge of diabetes adequate?*

Again, an answer based on your familiarity with the child may be adequate. However, if in doubt seek the advice of your pediatric endocrinologist.

MQ | *Is this youngster's emotional and social disposition up to the task?*

If the youngster tends to act out (to behave inappropriately or aggressively) when frustrated or discontent, be cautious. You may need professional guidance with this matter.

In most cases, the parents establish the foundation for what lies ahead. Parents who effectively manage their child's diabetes offer knowledgeable guidance, are not unduly emotional, and demonstrate good coping and adaptive skills. Doing the right things and doing them well over time serves as a model of behavior as the child becomes more independent and more prepared to take on some responsibility for his or her diabetes care. However, there are several deciding factors between knowing what to do and doing it: self-confidence, peer support versus bullying, disposition, and level of general contentment. There is no equation or test that would even approach this matter. The safest way to determine if children are ready to take on some degree of managing their diabetes is to consult with their medical team, their teachers, and the parents of their peers, who may observe the child's behavior in a less rigid environment.

CHALLENGE: SIBLINGS

The siblings of a child with diabetes may have the perception that the one with the ailment gets more attention than they do, and they may feel jealous and resentful. Seeing themselves as getting less attention might also be perceived as their being undeserving of parental love and devotion. Another danger for the siblings is the possibility that they will become fearful of developing diabetes themselves. Even classmates might misunderstand any extra attention the child with diabetes might receive in school.

Another potential problem for a sibling is the feeling of guilt for not having the disease. This feeling is analogous to a soldier returning from combat feeling guilty that he survived but a comrade had not come through their ordeal.

Parents and other caregivers need to use their eyes and ears to detect signs that a brother or sister is having a problem with regard to the sibling with diabetes. If you see signs of unexplainable irritability or distress, do not hesitate to ask if the youngster is upset. A child might be reticent and deny that there is a problem. If there are the slightest signs of discontent, continue to seek an understanding of what is happening in a manner that makes the youngster feel comfortable and safe.

Siblings may feel more connected and more valued if they have a part in the diabetes routine, perhaps helping to gather supplies both for checking the current blood glucose level and for administering a dose of insulin. Consider, too—for the sake of the youth with diabetes and any siblings—to attempt to make healthy choices as a family (e.g., everyone has the same snack or dinner rather than having something separate for the child with diabetes).

Consider these *mindful questions* directed at you and the son or daughter you are concerned about.

MQ | *Honey, it must be hard sometimes to see your brother/sister not feeling well (or seeing your mom so upset). It's OK. Can we just talk about it?*

Honey, I think you are upset. Can you tell me what is wrong?

Sweetheart, you do know how much daddy and I love you?

Do others—family members, other siblings, teachers, or peers—think that a sibling is troubled by the family situation?

Of course, the exact wording will vary with the age of the seemingly distressed child and the situation. The objective is to make the child feel safe in sharing with you. When a sibling denies to reveal some discontent that is seemingly apparent, it is time to go into problem-solving mode. (See Chapter 11: Problem Solving).

Sources of Stress for the Child With Type 1 Diabetes

For a child with type 1 diabetes, problems vary depending on the age at diagnosis. An infant might be momentarily agitated by an insulin injection or by a significant change in blood glucose levels, but a baby is not capable of being defiant or deliberately troublesome. From toddler to teenager, a range of attitudes and behaviors can make managing the diabetes difficult. A child with this disease can be feisty, even rebellious, again varying by age. Going through the stages of growth and development, children and their parents face different challenges. Adding diabetes or any chronic disease can make the journey much more challenging.

CHALLENGE: EMOTIONS

When an infant feels pain, the expression of discomfort and fear manifest in crying, along with flailing of arms and legs. Parents may feel a sense of pity, but the situation is usually resolved by offering the baby a pacifier and a hug. Managing diabetes becomes more complex as a child becomes increasingly independent. It doesn't take long for a baby to begin expressing discontent for reasons other than hunger or a messy diaper.

Children of preschool age are mostly, if not entirely, dependent on adults for their diabetes care. Unfortunately, the challenges for the parents and other care providers increase as the child develops. Toddlers (ages 1–3 years old) may forcefully object to their diabetes regimen. Preschool children (ages 3–5 years old) are no longer babies; they will almost surely exercise their increased independence, sometimes to the detriment of their diabetes regimen.

Diabetes management for school-age children (6–12 years old) can be difficult due, in part, to the increased interaction with their peers. Psychosocial and diabetes-related tension and stress for youngsters with diabetes generally begin at 7–8 years of age. Kids want to be a part of the group, not outsiders; this may lead to behavior that conflicts with effective diabetes management. An adolescent boy or girl may be persuaded to smoke cigarettes because of peer pressure. Youngsters with type 1 diabetes may be bullied for having authorization to leave the classroom or for getting special attention.

At this age, some youngsters show a degree of independence that can be problematic. For some, however, independence is favorable if it is used in positive ways, including recognizing the importance of managing diabetes.

Adolescence is the period from puberty to maturity, from childhood to adulthood. It is a time of turmoil generated by physical development, including the onset of puberty. In adolescence, there are dramatic changes both physical and mental, with the production of sex hormones, the maturing of the reproductive organs, and other sexual characteristics. These developments affect behavior and lifestyle.

Studies suggest that the changes in adolescence are associated with poor glycemic regulation. The causes of this decline include a decrease in the ability to self-manage the changes, the onset of menstruation, and increased insulin resistance in puberty. Also, the regimen may be disregarded because it interferes with other interests and activities. A teenagers' hormonal activity can play havoc with their physical and emotional state, which can be confusing and frustrating. Some juveniles rebel, tweaking their regimen despite the problems that follow. Once again, parents and other care providers are challenged by a range of issues that change as the child develops physically and emotionally.

Children with diabetes, especially in the latter stages of development, are prone to self-blame and believing that they are a burden to their family. Consequently, hearing their parents arguing about something totally unrelated to them can trigger undue feelings of guilt and shame. If a child witnesses an argument between parents, it is important to make it clear that the disagreement had nothing to do with him or her.

Mindful Solutions

From childhood to adulthood, the emotions and behavior of the youngster require patience, understanding, and, to a degree, acceptance of deviant behavior. Keep in mind that feistiness and rebelliousness are typical of all children as they grow, develop, and test boundaries. There are times when teenagers will outsmart and outshine their elders. But, in general, as mature as kids may appear, they are still kids. It is a fact that the human brain does not develop fully until the mid-20s.

Here are two stress-producing scenarios that might happen to a youngster with diabetes:

CHALLENGE: PARTY SCENE

Suppose your daughter comes home from an overnight pajama party and her blood glucose level was well above her target? Having had very little sleep, she was tired and decided to wait until she got home so you could inject her. This scenario would likely trigger negative emotions from a parent. *Living mindfully*, becoming aware of your unpleasant feelings, activates your *centering* process, followed by asking the following *mindful questions*:

MQ

I need to talk to my daughter about what happened. Would it be wise to give her time to settle down and, perhaps, to nap now? This would give me time to reflect on how to keep this from happening again. A good idea.

Did I overestimate her ability to manage her behavior or did I underestimate the potential distractions in that setting?

How can I prepare her for the next party event?

Did I not communicate adequately with the parents overseeing the party

> *regarding my daughter's diabetes-related issues?*
>
> *What do I need to do to be certain parents are fully informed regarding our child? Should I provide written guidelines?*

Let your daughter know that you understand the hardship imposed on her by the regimen for managing diabetes and the added burden of being in an unfamiliar situation. Lovingly express your concern for her safety and happiness. If she starts to cry, hold and comfort her; do not tell her she shouldn't cry. Compassion is primary in the pursuit of a positive outcome.

MQ | *Who can I ask for advice in this matter—someone in our support group or on our professional team?*

It can be very comforting to talk with someone who has been where you are now—perhaps a friend or a member of your support group. Pediatric care providers are a good source of advice regarding the challenges a child faces, such as undergoing peer pressure or having a sense of confusion in an unfamiliar setting.

CHALLENGE: SCHOOL SCENE

Imagine that your son came home from school in tears after some classmates teased and bullied him because a class had been interrupted when the teacher suspected that he was hypoglycemic. Realizing that you feel both helpless and infuriated, you take a moment to *center* followed by a series of *mindful questions*:

MQ | *How can I soothe his hurt feelings?*

Start by asking him what you can do to be helpful. Listen calmly, carefully, and compassionately. Because bullies feed off of the reactions of their victims, advise him to not react to their taunts and to walk away. Assure him that you know that wouldn't be easy to do, but that it can discourage their bullying. Although some adults might disagree, the best advice for a bullied child is, "Don't fight back." He or she should be advised to stay away from places where bullying happens. Staying near adults and other kids will lower the risk of being abused, since most bullying happens when adults aren't around.

> *MQ* | *What can I do to reframe this incident to make it an esteem-building opportunity?* (See Chapter 8: Reframing.)

If his frame is in the realm of, "I'm not good enough for them" or "I must deserve it," then the reframe could be, "These bullies are cowards who are so unhappy that they try to make others unhappy. This has nothing to do with who I am."

If bullying occurs, it is important to inform school officials and teachers as an immediate means of protecting your child from harm. Ideally, taking this step will increase the interest of encouraging a broader effort by the school and the community to resolve this and other potential problems. If, for example, students and their parents had a basic understanding of diabetes, they would more likely be empathetic and supportive of a classmate with the disease.

> *MQ* | *Should I petition the school to conduct a program to educate the students about bullying and about diabetes? Could I initiate the creation of a community-wide bullying prevention strategy?*

If I know the bullies' parents, should I talk to them and ask them to speak to their kids?

If you know the parents and have reason to believe that they will be understanding and empathetic, absolutely seek their help. Request that these parents approach their kids in a kindhearted manner and suggest that punishing them might give cause to bully your child again.

It Takes a Village

An aggregate of people is needed to effectively care for and raise a child with diabetes. A pediatric/diabetes team might start with a pediatrician or pediatric endocrinologist and a pediatric nurse. The American Diabetes Association recommends that mental health professionals should be an integral part of the team. As needed, other pediatric specialists would become involved.

CHALLENGES

Although it has been assumed that the primary caregivers are the child's parents, there are other scenarios—a single parent, grandparents or other family members, foster parents, or an agency having principle responsibility for the child's well-being. In each of these situations, the challenges are likely to be greater. A stay-at-home mom may be ill or she simply needs some time for herself. Grandparents may not be in good health or they simply might lack the energy required by the situation.

Having others available to backup primary caregivers is essential. As the child branches out socially and subsequently attends school, an adult needs to be present who recognizes and understands the signs of a problem and the steps to be taken to resolve it. When the youngster goes to a friend's birthday party, an adult should be present who knows the basics of type 1 diabetes. Although school nurses are well trained regarding this disease, it is essential that parents meet with nurses and teachers to scrutinize diabetes management needs. A medical management plan should be in place in school and updated periodically. The plan should include all of the necessary medical information for diabetes management in school.

In addition, a child who attends a school with federal funding has a right to a 504 plan to ensure appropriate accommodations are in place at the school. Section 504 of the Rehabilitation Act of 1973 sets out the actions the school will take to make sure the student with diabetes is medically safe, has the same access to education as other children, and is treated fairly. To become familiar with the plan and its numerous provisions, go to the American Diabetes Association's website, diabetes.org, and enter "Section 504 plan" in the search box near the top right corner of the page. A new page will appear with the link to the 504 plan near the top.

While social support is important both for the child and the parents, care must be taken that designated supporters are well-informed and reliable. The literature suggests that what may appear to be a source of support can hinder the management of the disease. Grandma or Aunt Sarah should know that the regimen for managing the disease is necessary for the youngster's well-being. They should understand that he or she can have a moderate portion of cake and ice cream with everyone else, but being overly sympathetic and allowing the child to overindulge could have unpleasant consequences.

Trustworthy supporters will reduce the stress imposed on primary providers of a child with diabetes. Having others "on the team" will minimize feelings of isolation and despair, especially in difficult times.

If there is a support group nearby—even if it is not intended specifically for type 1 diabetes—be open-minded and give it a try for two reasons. First, there are factors regarding living with diabetes that are as relevant for a senior adult as for a teenager and as meaningful with either type 1 or type 2 diabetes. Second, the emotional support and compassion of fellow "travelers" can be priceless.

Do not hesitate to seek the assistance of the child's professional care providers. This step may seem obvious, but some individuals are hesitant to call for help, believing it would be an imposition or it somehow would be unacceptable. If you are concerned about what is happening and you don't know what to do, call the doctor, nurse educator, or diabetes center for help. In the unlikely event that someone is annoyed by your call, it is their problem not yours. And before you call or seek direct help, make a list of your concerns and questions. Under stress, you are likely to forget something that is important.

As always, when circumstances are important and complex, ask the *mindful questions*:

MQ | *Which family members and friends might be willing and able to provide support for our child?*

Are they willing to take the time to learn the basics of diabetes management and issues specific to our child?

Is there any reason to doubt their reliability?

Getting answers to these three questions will help you determine anyone's trustworthiness. If they are enthusiastic about helping you but you have concern about their reliability, do not enlist their support. It wouldn't be worth the risk.

MQ | *Do we have a plan for the support person(s) and me to communicate, if necessary?*

Given the prevalence of cell phones, being able to connect should be easy. Because a variety of ringtones are available on smartphones, consider choosing one that immediately alerts you that the person caring for your child is calling.

Most people are good-hearted and well-intentioned. Given the stakes in caring for a young child with diabetes, it is reasonable to be guarded to the extent of asking the *mindful questions* before placing your youngster in someone's care.

The vast majority of children diagnosed with type 1 diabetes are able to bear the trials and tribulations imposed by the disease. Although the learning curve for adjusting and coping to the ailment resets with age and stages of development, most children are able to do well in the long run when given proper attention, care, and guidance.

Ultimately, success in raising a child with type 1 diabetes depends primarily on the parents or primary adult care providers. The more they are diabetes smart, emotionally steady, and have a balance between sturdiness and tolerance, the better. Of course, a diabetes-oriented medical team is essential. Websites offer useful information and advice but cannot replace the need for direct medical attention (see Chapter 14: The Internet: Excellent with Caution). A solid, well-informed support system plays a vital role in reducing the stress imposed on the primary care providers.

Raising a child with diabetes can be described as an adventure. It is a journey over time that includes the unknown, both pleasant and unpleasant surprises, danger, excitement, unexpected problems, disappointments, and rewards. Unfortunately, it is human nature to become so enmeshed in the negatives that we are deaf and blind to the positives. I am reminded of a card on my desk with the words of Vivian Greene that says, "Life isn't about waiting for the storm to pass. It's about learning how to dance in the rain."

Living *mindfully* is empowering. It is the ideal mindset for minimizing stress and maximizing self-control. *Mindfulness* counteracts self-defeating behaviors like being locked into pessimism, helplessness, or hopelessness. A practice of *mindfulness* neither exaggerates nor underestimates the seriousness of a situation. Living *mindfully* makes the adventure exactly as it is—no less, no more.

PART 5

*Final Thoughts
and Resources*

AFTERWORD

I do not have diabetes. I have coronary artery disease and had triple bypass surgery in 1993. Although diabetes is more challenging to manage, there are significant similarities between these diseases. I cannot eat everything I want or as much as I want sometimes. I wish I could stop exercising because it is very tiring at my age, but I can't. I have to take medications that require me to have an insurance plan that is very costly. There are so many ways that stress can be harmful to my vascular system and heart.

The bad news: my disease and yours need continual commitment, discipline, patience, hope, and a lot of smarts. Oh, and I almost forgot. They also require the fortitude and resilience to bounce back from the falls that are inevitable.

The good news: being mindful gives us the power to manage our medical conditions effectively despite their many demands and inhibitions. A mindful approach is a powerful way to manage the stress demons of disease. Living mindfully keeps us informed of what is working and what is not going well. When we are aware of what we are thinking, feeling, and doing, we are aware, too, of the *mindful questions* that serve as a mental compass, leading us in the right direction.

When mindlessness was my natural way, I might have realized I was in a bad place hours or days after suffering over something, and even then, it might not have occurred to me that I had other choices that might spare me more distress. Living mindlessly is an open invitation to stress and misfortune.

Reflecting on *mindful questions* opens a range of possibilities for changing something that isn't working into something that does work. The process of mindfulness enables us to choose from many options—reframing faulty beliefs, outsmarting our feelings, shifting into problem-solving mode, laughing at our foibles, and many more—that empower us to keep the stresses of disease and life in check.

In *The Choice* (17), Og Mandino wrote, *"Those who live in unhappy failure have never exercised their options for a better way of life because they have never been aware that they had any choices."*

While reframing a faulty belief is a powerful stress-buster, it is even better to start with a positive frame and eliminate the need for reframing. Here are some frames that have worked for me:

- I have everything I need to do what is needed to get where I want to be.
- One day at a time; sometimes, one moment at a time.
- When something doesn't work for me twice, it really gets my attention.
- I choose not to let others steal my worth or time.
- Anything meaningless in the face of death is meaningless.
- I don't believe everything I think.
- Everything that happens to me is fascinating . . . well, almost everything.

You have everything you need to minimize the stress of diabetes and life—everything to maximize your ability to manage diabetes well. Whether it will happen or not depends on your commitment to practice the principles and skills that have been presented in this book. It is fitting to conclude with a comment by one of the greatest coaches in football history, Vince Lombardi: *"The only place you'll find success before work is in the dictionary."*

Mastering the fundamentals of mindfulness is work, and developing the ability to live mindfully is work; it is the path to success in mastering the stress that is a principal nemesis of diabetes management. Get to work.

RESOURCES

References

1. Napora JP. *Stress-Free Diabetes: Your Guide to Health and Happiness.* Arlington, VA, American Diabetes Association, 2010

2. Heschel AJ. *Man Is Not Alone: A Philosophy of Religion.* New York, Farrar, Straus, and Giroux, 1951

3. Newberg A, Waldman MR. *Why We Believe What We Believe: Uncovering Our Biological Need for Meaning, Spirituality, and Truth.* New York, Free Press, 2006

4. Buettner D. *The Blue Zones: Lessons for Living Longer from the People Who've Lived the Longest.* Washington, DC, National Geographic Society, 2008

5. Dalai Lama, Cutler HC. *The Art of Happiness: A Handbook for Living.* New York, Riverhead Books, 1988

6. Frankl V. *Man's Search for Meaning.* Boston, MA, Beacon Press, 1962

7. Beisser AB. *Flying Without Wings.* New York, Bantam Books, 1990

8. Lamott A. *Traveling Mercies.* New York, Pantheon, 1999

9. Johnson S. *Who Moved My Cheese?* New York, Putnam, 1998

10. Zander RS, Zander B. *The Art of Possibility: Transforming Professional and Personal Life.* Boston, MA, Harvard Business School Press, 2000

11. Rizzo A. Father Rizzo Speaks. Monograph. 1980

12. Walsh JJ. *Laughter and Health.* New York, Appleton, 1928

13. Cousins N. *Anatomy of an Illness.* New York, Norton, 1979

14. Napora JP. *A Study of the Effects of a Program of Humorous Activity on the Subjective Well-Being of Senior Adults.* PhD thesis. Baltimore, MD, University of Maryland School of Social Work, 1984

15. Rubin RR, Biermann J, Toohey B. *Psyching Out Diabetes: A Positive Approach to Your Negative Emotions.* Los Angeles, CA, Lowell House, 1992

16. Kabat-Zinn J. *Full Catastrophe Living: Using the Wisdom of Your Body and Mind to Face Stress, Pain, and Illness.* New York, Dell, 2005

17. Mandino O. *The Choice.* New York, Bantam Press, 1984

Suggested Readings

American Diabetes Association. *Managing Type 2 Diabetes for Dummies.* Hoboken, NJ, John Wiley & Sons, 2018

Arsham G, Lowe E. *Diabetes: A Guide to Living Well.* 4th ed. Alexandria, VA, American Diabetes Association, 2004

Benson H, Klipper MZ. *The Relaxation Response.* New York, Avon, 1976

Fox LA, Weber SL. *Diabetes 911: How to Handle Everyday Emergencies.* Alexandria, VA, American Diabetes Association, 2009

Gorman SE, Gorman JM. *Denying to the Grave: Why We Ignore the Facts that Will Save Us.* New York, Oxford University Press, 2017

Hoff B. *The Tao of Pooh.* New York, Penguin Books, 1983

Kabat-Zinn J. *Wherever You Go, There You Are.* New York, Hyperion, 1994

Plumb C. *I'm No Hero.* Mechanicsburg, PA, Executive Press, 1973

Sapolsky RM. *Why Zebras Don't Get Ulcers.* New York, W.H. Freeman, 1998

Saudek CD, Rubin RR, Donner TW. *The Johns Hopkins Guide to Diabetes: For Patients and Family.* Baltimore, MD, Johns Hopkins Press, 2014

Selye H. *The Stress of Life.* New York, McGraw-Hill, 1956

Selye H. *Stress Without Distress.* Philadelphia, Lippincott, 1974

Watts AW. *The Wisdom of Insecurity.* New York, Vintage Books, 1961

Wood J, Peters A. *The Type 1 Diabetes Self-Care Manual: A Complete Guide to Type 1 Diabetes Across the Lifespan for People with Diabetes, Parents, and Caregivers.* Alexandria, VA, American Diabetes Association, 2017

Recommended Diabetes-Related Websites and Apps

diabeteseducator.org (American Association of Diabetes Educators [AADE])

diabetes.org (American Diabetes Association)

healthfinder.gov (Office of Disease Prevention and Health Promotion in the U.S. Department of Health and Human Services)

joslin.org (Joslin Diabetes Center)

medlineplus.com (National Library of Medicine, National Institutes of Health)

niddk.nih.gov (National Institute of Diabetes and Digestive and Kidney Diseases [NIDDK])

Recommended Podcasts

- diabetesdoingthings.com
  - Thirty-minute candid conversations with "everyday" people dealing with type 1 diabetes.
- diabetes-connections.com
  - The mother of a son with type 1 diabetes shares personal anecdotes and interviews with fellow diabetes advocates.
- diabetesdailygrind.com/real-life-diabetes
  - Blog features guests who share fresh ideas about diabetes management.
- ontrackdiabetes.com/all-webinars-podcasts
  - Episodes cover a variety of subjects for people with type 1 diabetes, type 2 diabetes, and prediabetes.
- blogtalkradio.com/divatalkradio1
  - The host chats with care providers and beauty and style experts affected by diabetes.
- ardensday.com (The Juicebox Podcast)
  - A series of conversations between people grappling with their diagnosis or that of a loved one.
- soundbitesrd.com
  - A registered dietitian interviews researchers, nutritionists, and dietitians about meal-planning issues.

- diabetesjournals.org/content/diabetes-core-update-podcasts
  - The American Diabetes Association presents an in-depth look at recently published scholarly articles that are "easily digestible" for anyone interested in the latest diabetes developments.

Recommended General Health Websites

www.ama-assn.org (American Medical Association)

www.kidshealth.org (Kids Health)

www.mayoclinic.com (Mayo Clinic)

https://www.nia.nih.gov (National Institute on Aging)

www.nih.gov (National Institutes of Health)

www.nlm.nih.gov/medlineplus (National Library of Medicine, MedlinePlus)

Index